ULTIMATE FITNESS JOURNAL

for the Die-hard Fitness Enthusiast

Activinotes

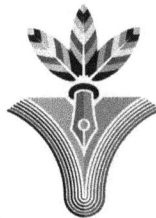

Activinotes

DAILY JOURNALS, PLANNERS, NOTEBOOKS AND OTHER BLANK BOOKS

Copyright 2016

DATE: _____ / _____ / _____

STRENGTH TRAINING   Time Start: Time Stop:

EXERCISE	SET 1	SET 2	SET 3	SET 4	SET5

CARDIO   Time Start: Time Stop:

EXERCISE	TIME	INTENSITY	DISTANCE	RATE	CALORIES

NOTES

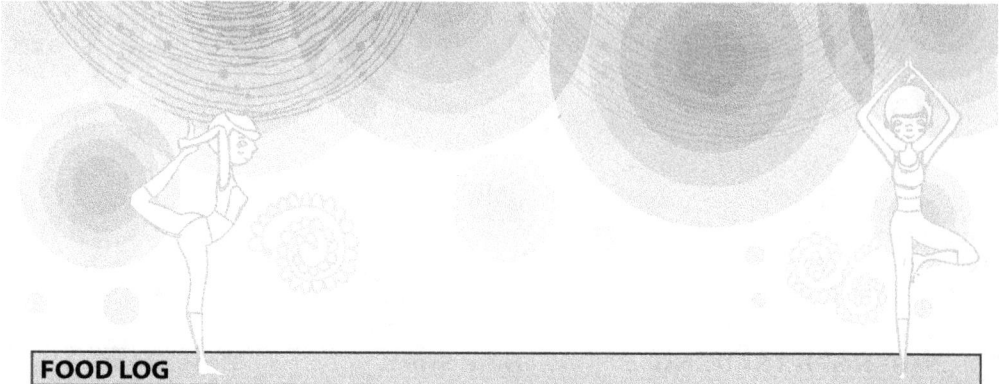

FOOD LOG

BREAKFAST	NOTES

SNACK	NOTES

LUNCH	NOTES

SNACK	NOTES

DINNER	NOTES

NUTRIENT TRACKER

	# OF SERVINGS						
GRAIN							
VEGGIES							
FRUITS							
DAIRY							
PROTEIN							
FATS							
VITAMINS							
SUGAR							

HOURS OF SLEEP: _____
GLASSES OF WATER FOR TODAY : _____

NOTES

What I have achieved Today

_____

_____

_____

_____

_____

What I need to improve next

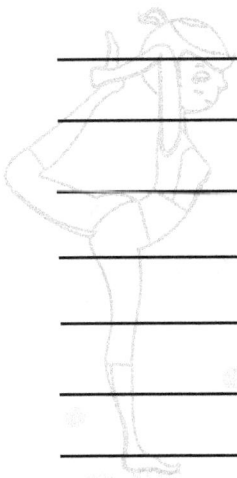

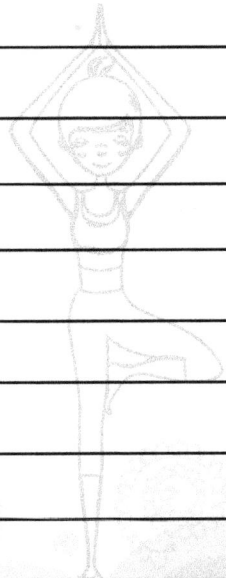

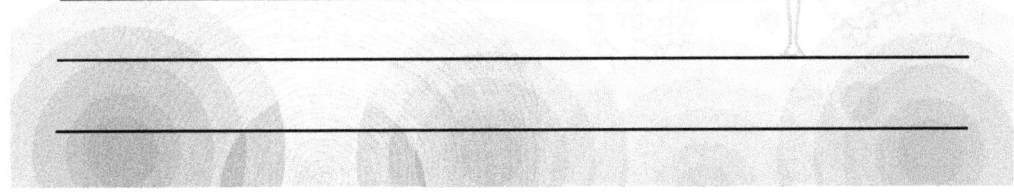

_____

_____

_____

_____

_____

_____

_____

_____

_____

_____

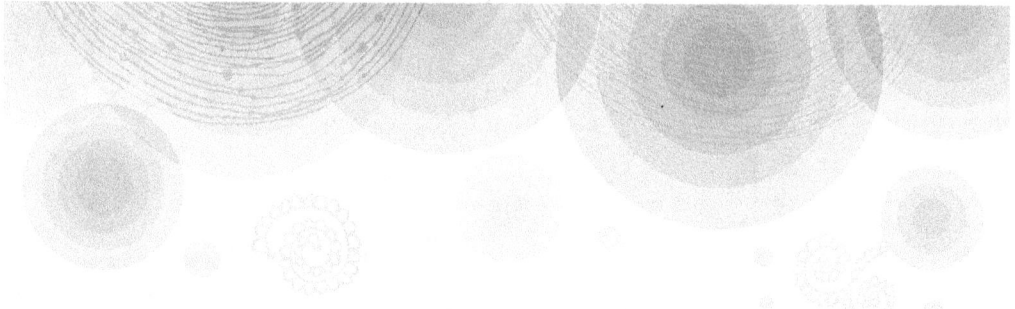

DATE: _____ / _____ / _____

STRENGTH TRAINING		Time Start:			Time Stop:	
EXERCISE	SET 1	SET 2	SET 3	SET 4	SET5

CARDIO		Time Start:		Time Stop:		
EXERCISE	TIME	INTENSITY	DISTANCE	RATE	CALORIES

NOTES

FOOD LOG

BREAKFAST	NOTES

SNACK	NOTES

LUNCH	NOTES

SNACK	NOTES

DINNER	NOTES

NUTRIENT TRACKER

	# OF SERVINGS						
GRAIN							
VEGGIES							
FRUITS							
DAIRY							
PROTEIN							
FATS							
VITAMINS							
SUGAR							

NOTES

HOURS OF SLEEP: _____
GLASSES OF WATER FOR TODAY : _____

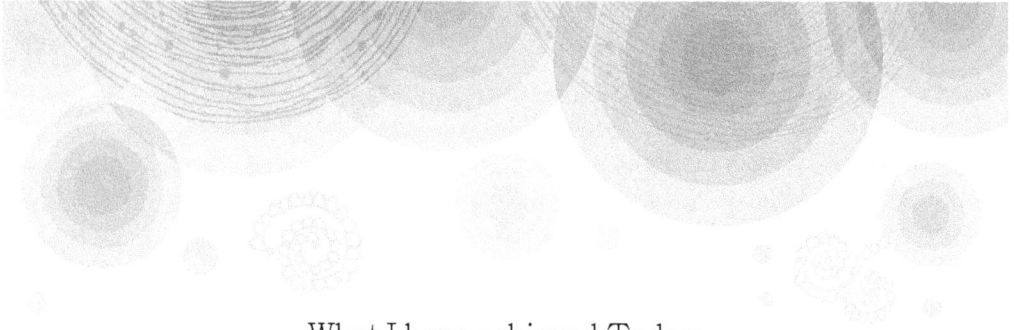

What I have achieved Today

_____

_____

_____

_____

_____

What I need to improve next

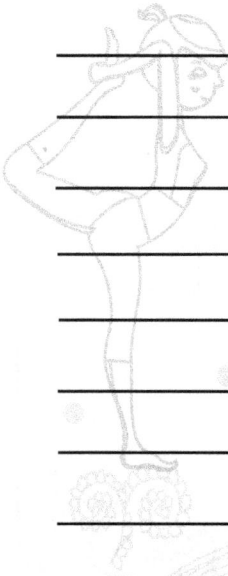

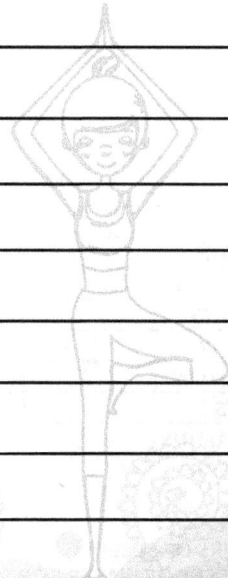

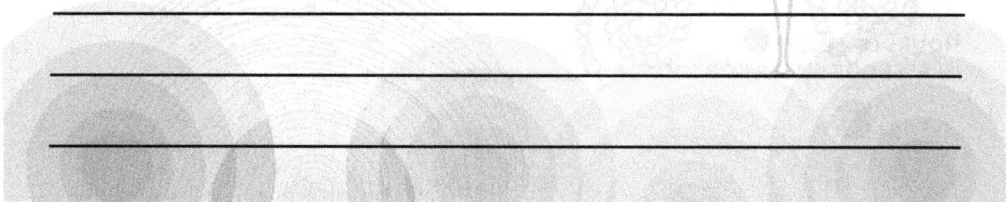

_____

_____

_____

_____

_____

_____

_____

_____

_____

DATE: _____ / _____ / _____

STRENGTH TRAINING	Time Start:		Time Stop:		
EXERCISE	SET 1	SET 2	SET 3	SET 4	SET5

CARDIO	Time Start:		Time Stop:		
EXERCISE	TIME	INTENSITY	DISTANCE	RATE	CALORIES

NOTES

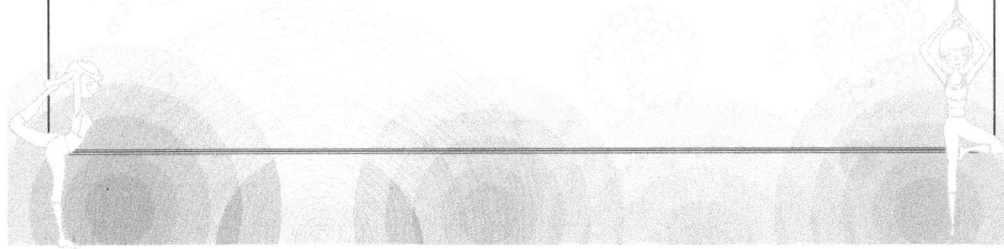

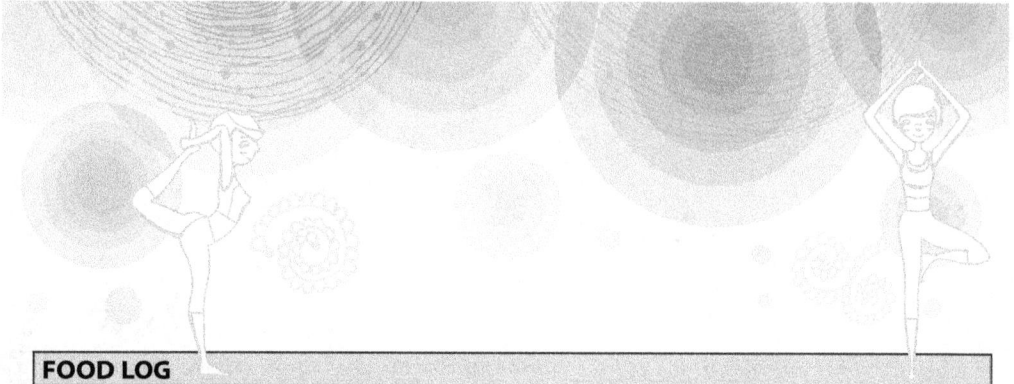

FOOD LOG

BREAKFAST	NOTES

SNACK	NOTES

LUNCH	NOTES

SNACK	NOTES

DINNER	NOTES

NUTRIENT TRACKER

	# OF SERVINGS						
GRAIN							
VEGGIES							
FRUITS							
DAIRY							
PROTEIN							
FATS							
VITAMINS							
SUGAR							

NOTES

HOURS OF SLEEP: _____

GLASSES OF WATER FOR TODAY : _____

What I have achieved Today

_____

_____

_____

_____

_____

_____

What I need to improve next

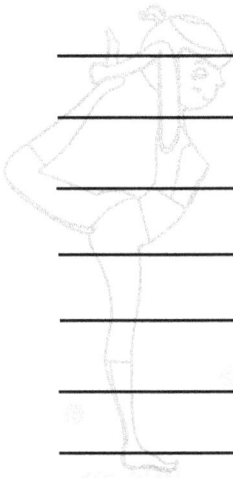

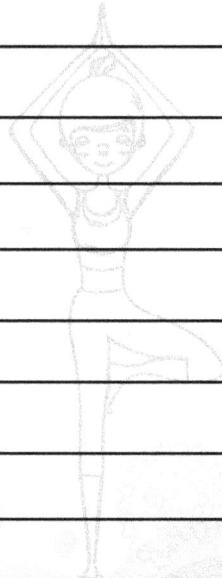

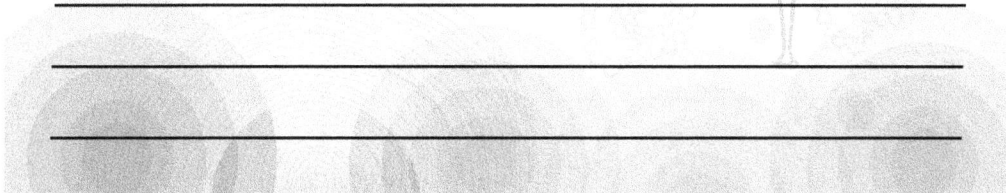

_____

_____

_____

_____

_____

_____

_____

_____

_____

DATE: _____ / _____ / _____

STRENGTH TRAINING	Time Start:		Time Stop:		
EXERCISE	SET 1	SET 2	SET 3	SET 4	SET5

CARDIO	Time Start:		Time Stop:		
EXERCISE	TIME	INTENSITY	DISTANCE	RATE	CALORIES

NOTES

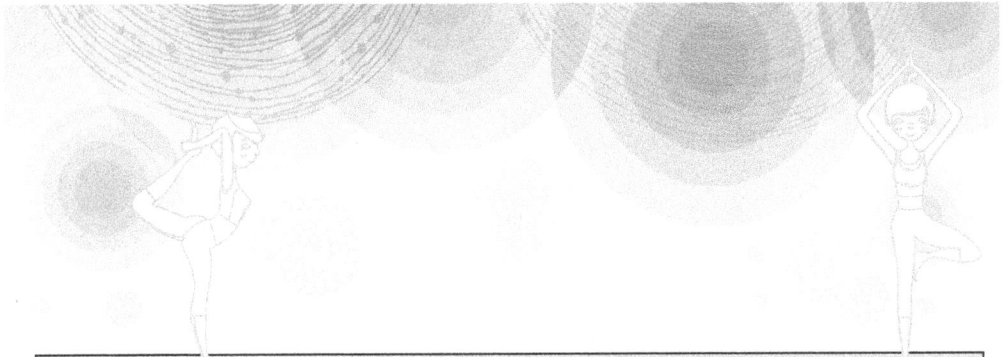

FOOD LOG

BREAKFAST	NOTES

SNACK	NOTES

LUNCH	NOTES

SNACK	NOTES

DINNER	NOTES

NUTRIENT TRACKER

	# OF SERVINGS						
GRAIN							
VEGGIES							
FRUITS							
DAIRY							
PROTEIN							
FATS							
VITAMINS							
SUGAR							

NOTES

HOURS OF SLEEP: _____
GLASSES OF WATER FOR TODAY : _____

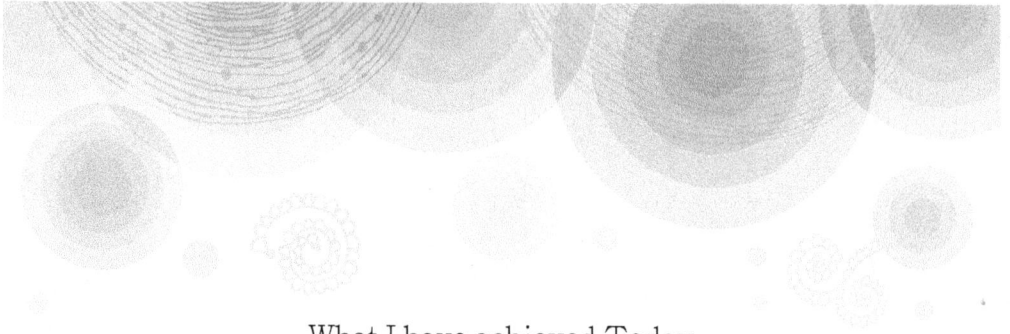

What I have achieved Today

_____

_____

_____

_____

_____

_____

What I need to improve next

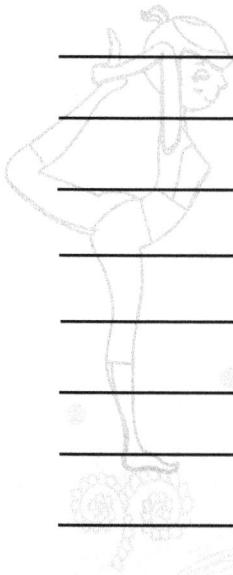

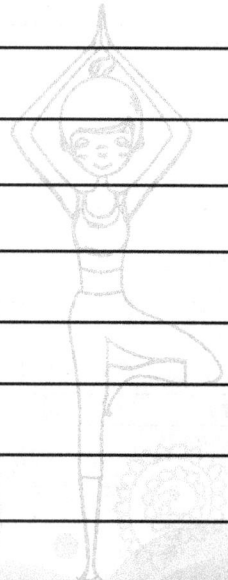

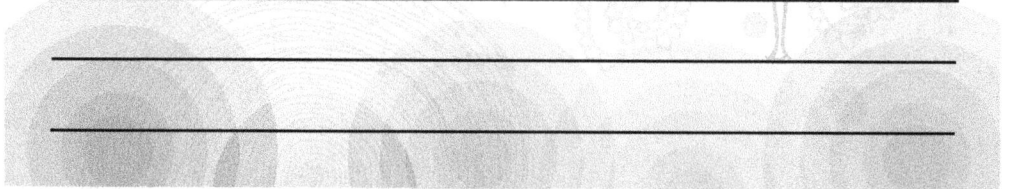

_____

_____

_____

_____

_____

_____

_____

_____

_____

_____

DATE: _____ / _____ / _____

STRENGTH TRAINING		Time Start:			Time Stop:	
EXERCISE	SET 1	SET 2	SET 3	SET 4	SET5

CARDIO		Time Start:			Time Stop:	
EXERCISE	TIME	INTENSITY	DISTANCE	RATE	CALORIES

NOTES

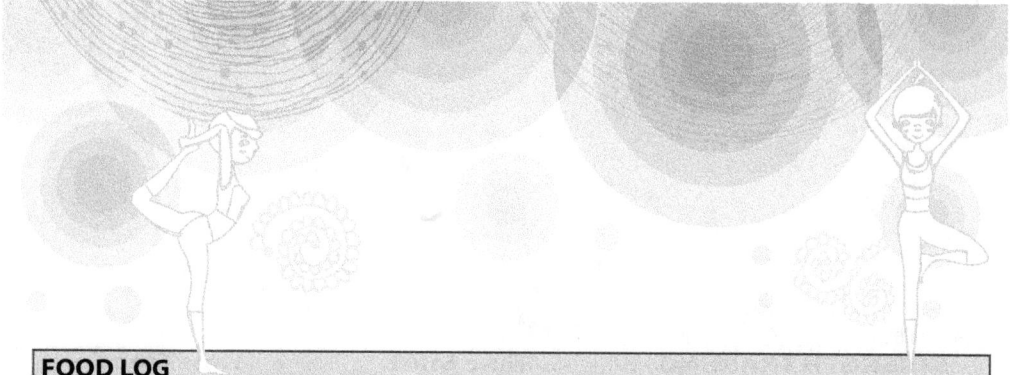

FOOD LOG

BREAKFAST	NOTES

SNACK	NOTES

LUNCH	NOTES

SNACK	NOTES

DINNER	NOTES

NUTRIENT TRACKER

	# OF SERVINGS						
GRAIN							
VEGGIES							
FRUITS							
DAIRY							
PROTEIN							
FATS							
VITAMINS							
SUGAR							

NOTES

HOURS OF SLEEP: _____
GLASSES OF WATER FOR TODAY : _____

What I have achieved Today

_____

_____

_____

_____

_____

What I need to improve next

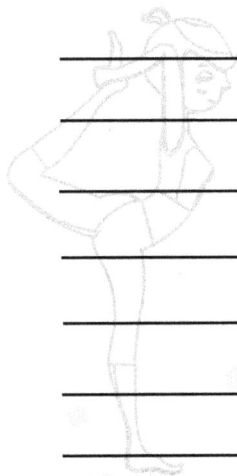

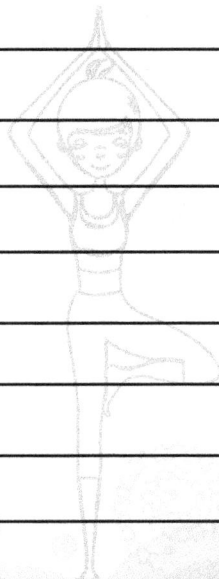

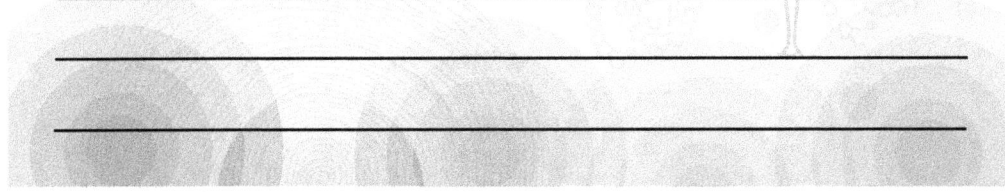

_____

_____

_____

_____

_____

_____

_____

_____

_____

DATE: _____/_____/_____

STRENGTH TRAINING		Time Start:		Time Stop:		
EXERCISE	SET 1	SET 2	SET 3	SET 4	SET5

CARDIO		Time Start:		Time Stop:		
EXERCISE	TIME	INTENSITY	DISTANCE	RATE	CALORIES

NOTES

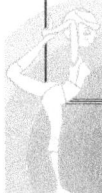
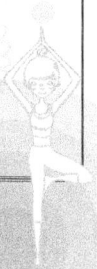

FOOD LOG

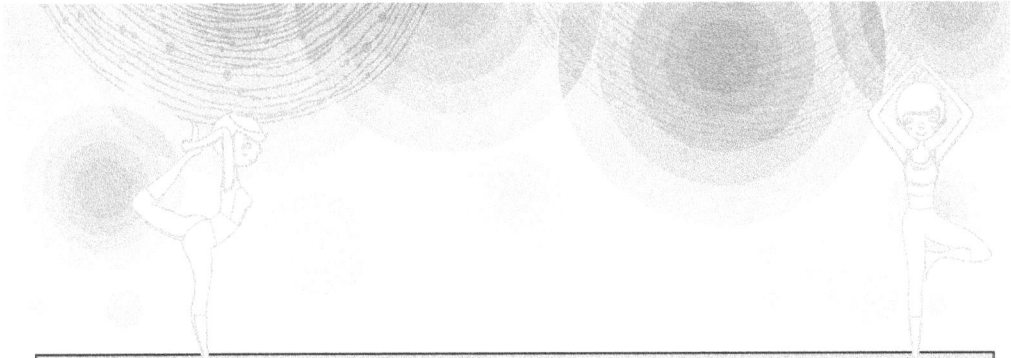

BREAKFAST	NOTES
SNACK	NOTES
LUNCH	NOTES
SNACK	NOTES
DINNER	NOTES

NUTRIENT TRACKER

	# OF SERVINGS						
GRAIN							
VEGGIES							
FRUITS							
DAIRY							
PROTEIN							
FATS							
VITAMINS							
SUGAR							

NOTES

HOURS OF SLEEP: _____

GLASSES OF WATER FOR TODAY : _____

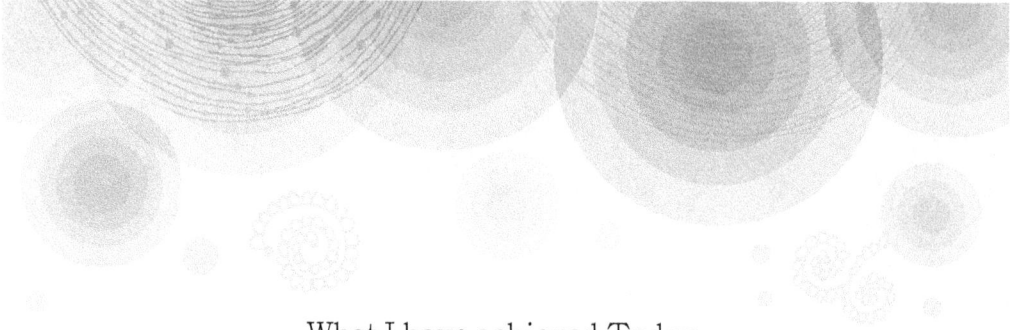

What I have achieved Today

_____

_____

_____

_____

_____

What I need to improve next

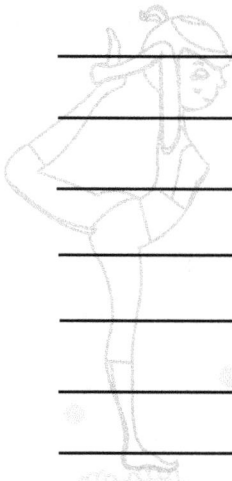

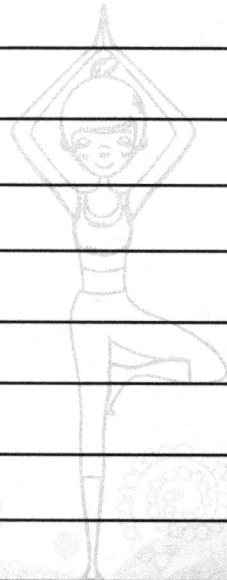

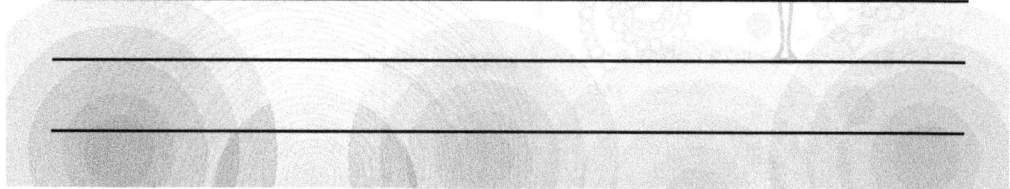

_____

_____

_____

_____

_____

_____

_____

_____

_____

DATE: _____/_____/_____

STRENGTH TRAINING	Time Start:		Time Stop:		
EXERCISE	SET 1	SET 2	SET 3	SET 4	SET5

CARDIO	Time Start:		Time Stop:		
EXERCISE	TIME	INTENSITY	DISTANCE	RATE	CALORIES

NOTES

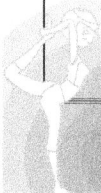
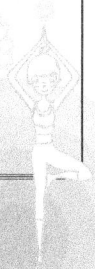

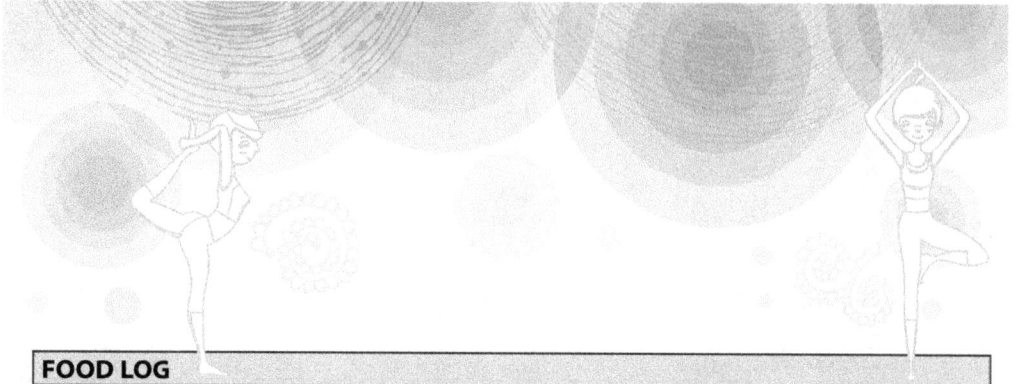

FOOD LOG

BREAKFAST	NOTES

SNACK	NOTES

LUNCH	NOTES

SNACK	NOTES

DINNER	NOTES

NUTRIENT TRACKER

	# OF SERVINGS						
GRAIN							
VEGGIES							
FRUITS							
DAIRY							
PROTEIN							
FATS							
VITAMINS							
SUGAR							

NOTES

HOURS OF SLEEP: _____
GLASSES OF WATER FOR TODAY : _____

What I have achieved Today

_____

_____

_____

_____

_____

_____

What I need to improve next

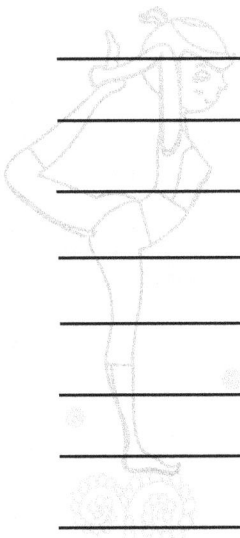

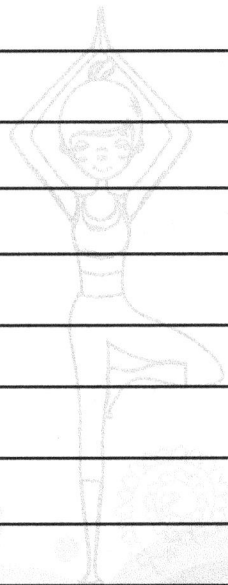

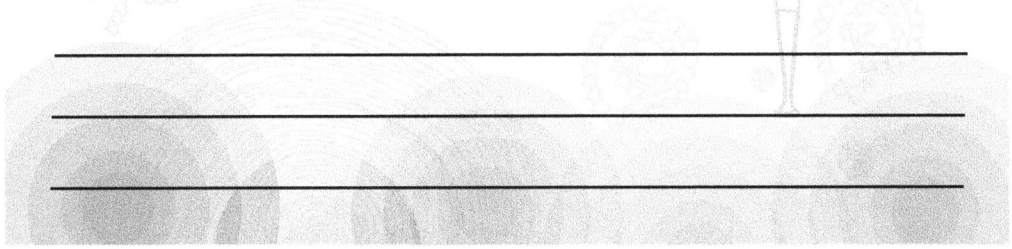

_____

_____

_____

_____

_____

_____

_____

_____

_____

_____

DATE: _____ / _____ / _____

STRENGTH TRAINING	Time Start:		Time Stop:		
EXERCISE	SET 1	SET 2	SET 3	SET 4	SET5

CARDIO	Time Start:		Time Stop:		
EXERCISE	TIME	INTENSITY	DISTANCE	RATE	CALORIES

NOTES

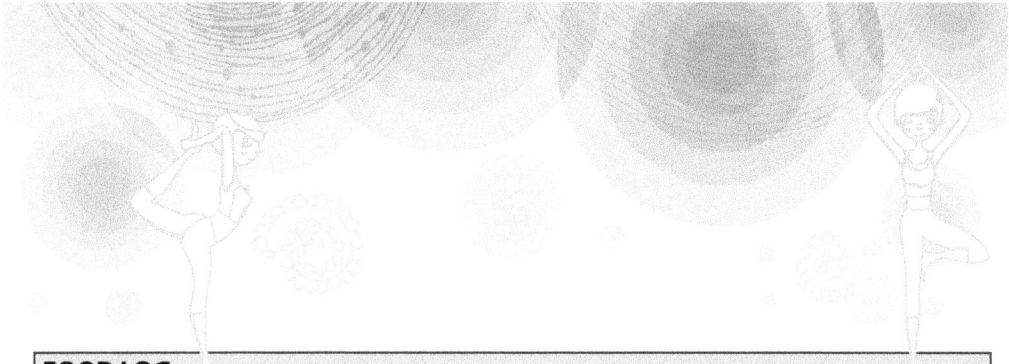

FOOD LOG

BREAKFAST	NOTES

SNACK	NOTES

LUNCH	NOTES

SNACK	NOTES

DINNER	NOTES

NUTRIENT TRACKER

	# OF SERVINGS						
GRAIN							
VEGGIES							
FRUITS							
DAIRY							
PROTEIN							
FATS							
VITAMINS							
SUGAR							

NOTES

HOURS OF SLEEP: _____
GLASSES OF WATER FOR TODAY : _____

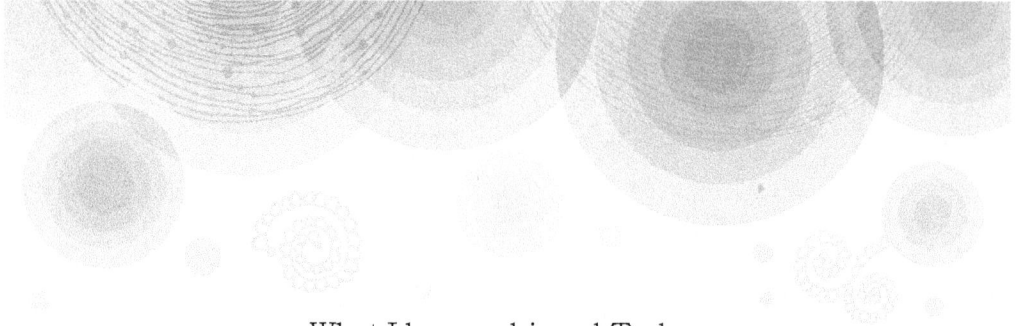

What I have achieved Today

_____

_____

_____

_____

_____

_____

What I need to improve next

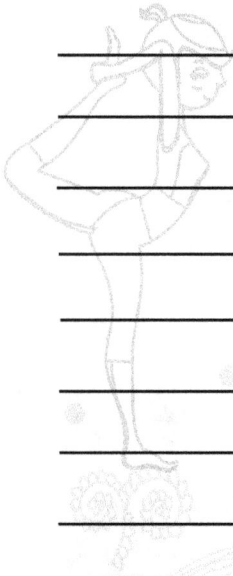

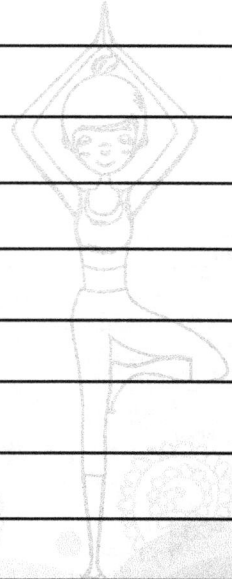

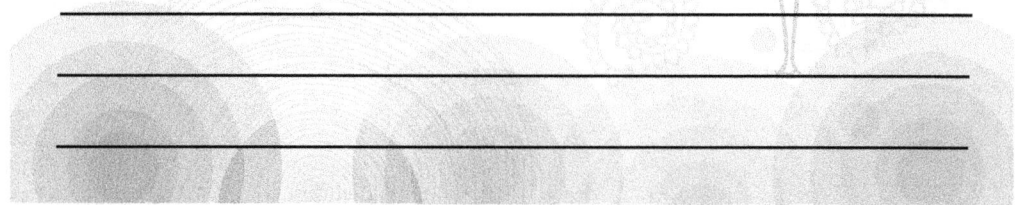

_____

_____

_____

_____

_____

_____

_____

_____

_____

_____

DATE: _____ / _____ / _____

STRENGTH TRAINING		Time Start:			Time Stop:	
EXERCISE	SET 1	SET 2	SET 3	SET 4	SET5

CARDIO		Time Start:		Time Stop:		
EXERCISE	TIME	INTENSITY	DISTANCE	RATE	CALORIES

NOTES

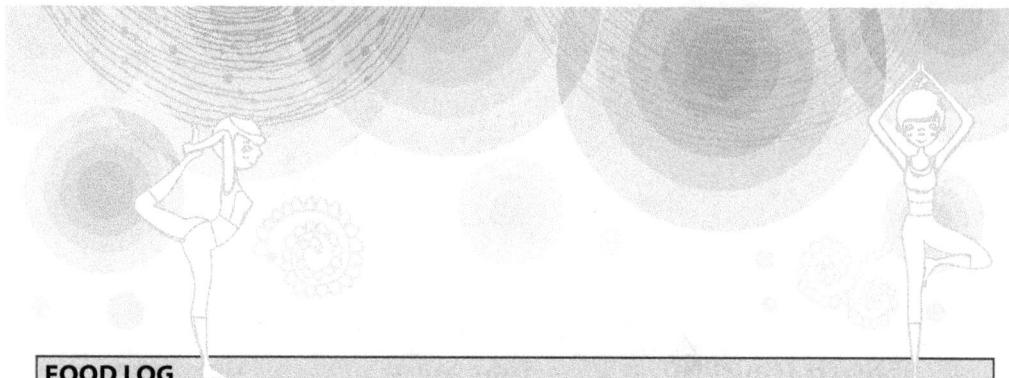

FOOD LOG

BREAKFAST	NOTES

SNACK	NOTES

LUNCH	NOTES

SNACK	NOTES

DINNER	NOTES

NUTRIENT TRACKER

	# OF SERVINGS						
GRAIN							
VEGGIES							
FRUITS							
DAIRY							
PROTEIN							
FATS							
VITAMINS							
SUGAR							

NOTES

HOURS OF SLEEP: _____

GLASSES OF WATER FOR TODAY : _____

What I have achieved Today

_____

_____

_____

_____

_____

What I need to improve next

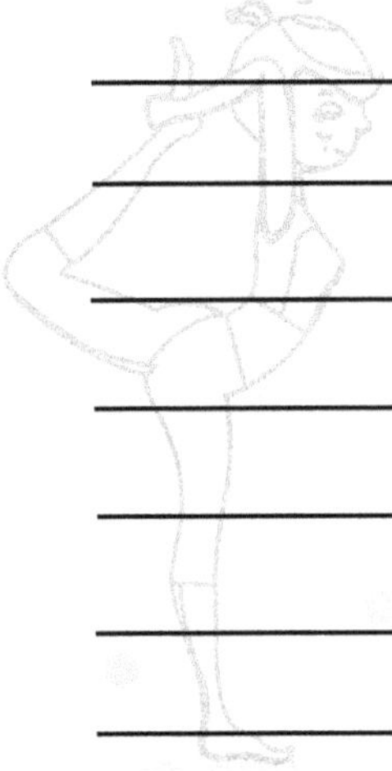

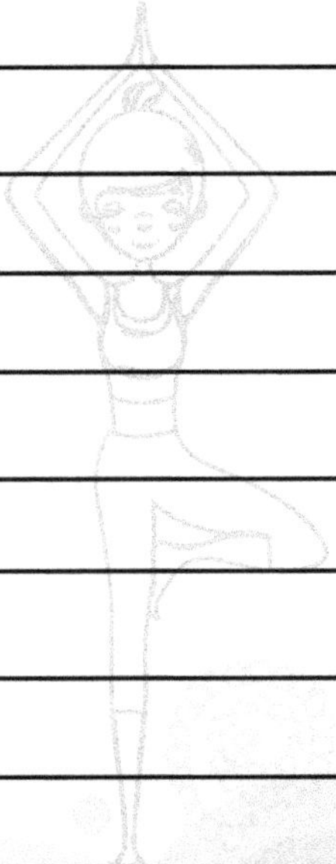

_____

_____

_____

_____

_____

_____

_____

_____

_____

_____

DATE: _____/_____/_____

STRENGTH TRAINING		Time Start:		Time Stop:		
EXERCISE		SET 1	SET 2	SET 3	SET 4	SET5

CARDIO	Time Start:		Time Stop:		
EXERCISE	TIME	INTENSITY	DISTANCE	RATE	CALORIES

NOTES

FOOD LOG

BREAKFAST	NOTES

SNACK	NOTES

LUNCH	NOTES

SNACK	NOTES

DINNER	NOTES

NUTRIENT TRACKER

	# OF SERVINGS						
GRAIN							
VEGGIES							
FRUITS							
DAIRY							
PROTEIN							
FATS							
VITAMINS							
SUGAR							

NOTES

HOURS OF SLEEP: _____

GLASSES OF WATER FOR TODAY : _____

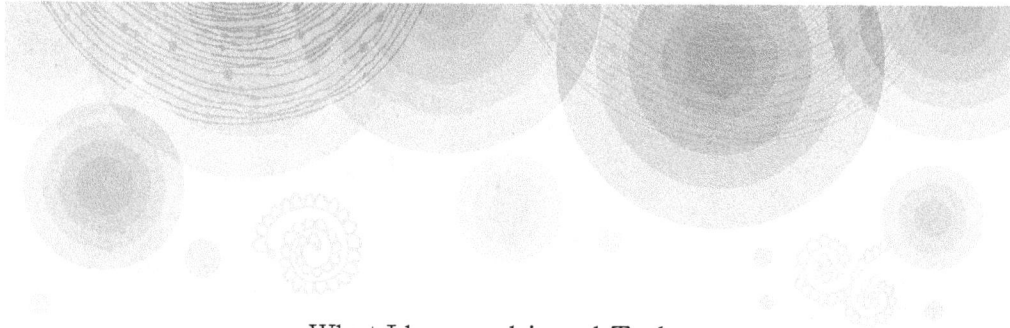

What I have achieved Today

_____

_____

_____

_____

_____

What I need to improve next

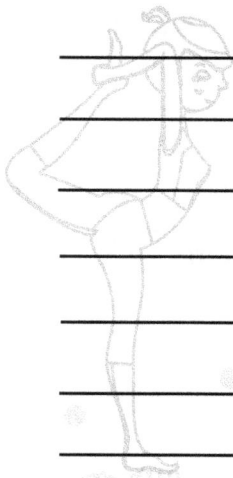

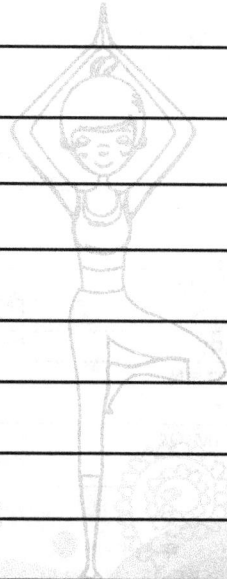

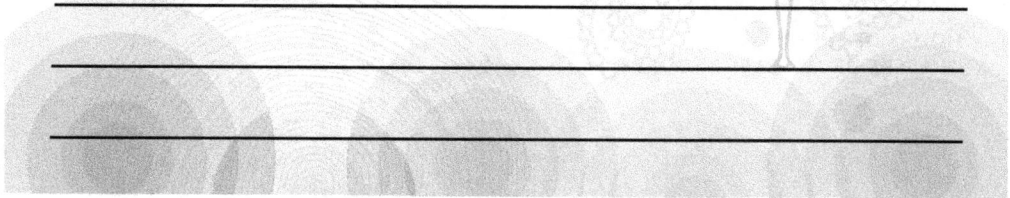

_____

_____

_____

_____

_____

_____

_____

_____

_____

DATE: _____/ _____/ _____

STRENGTH TRAINING   Time Start: Time Stop:

EXERCISE	SET 1	SET 2	SET 3	SET 4	SET5

CARDIO   Time Start: Time Stop:

EXERCISE	TIME	INTENSITY	DISTANCE	RATE	CALORIES

NOTES

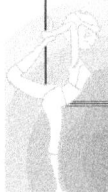
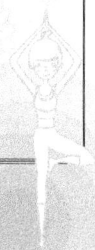

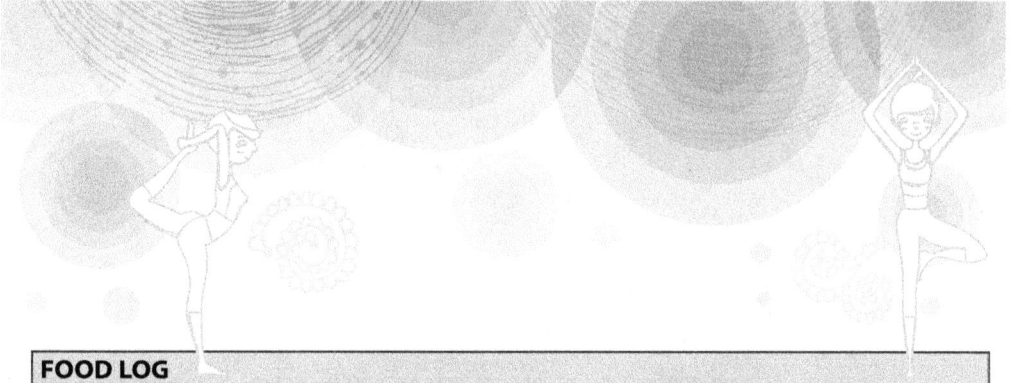

FOOD LOG

BREAKFAST	NOTES

SNACK	NOTES

LUNCH	NOTES

SNACK	NOTES

DINNER	NOTES

NUTRIENT TRACKER

	# OF SERVINGS						
GRAIN							
VEGGIES							
FRUITS							
DAIRY							
PROTEIN							
FATS							
VITAMINS							
SUGAR							

NOTES

HOURS OF SLEEP: _____
GLASSES OF WATER FOR TODAY : _____

What I have achieved Today

_____

_____

_____

_____

_____

_____

What I need to improve next

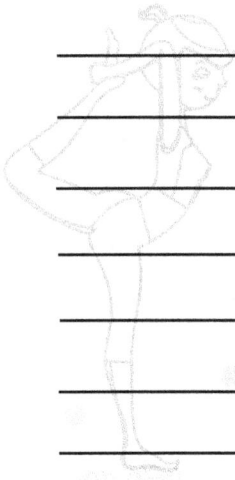

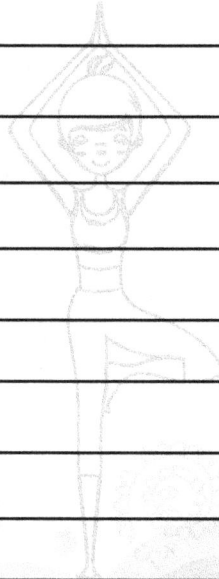

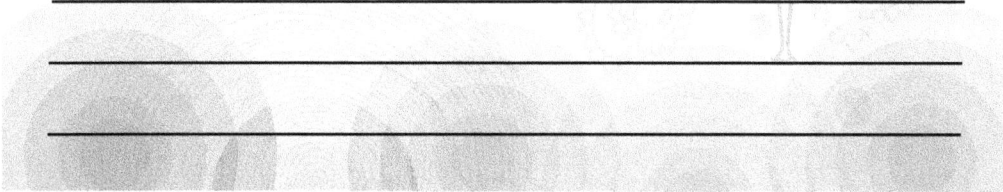

_____

_____

_____

_____

_____

_____

_____

_____

_____

_____

DATE: _____ / _____ / _____

STRENGTH TRAINING	Time Start:			Time Stop:	
EXERCISE	SET 1	SET 2	SET 3	SET 4	SET5

CARDIO	Time Start:		Time Stop:		
EXERCISE	TIME	INTENSITY	DISTANCE	RATE	CALORIES

NOTES

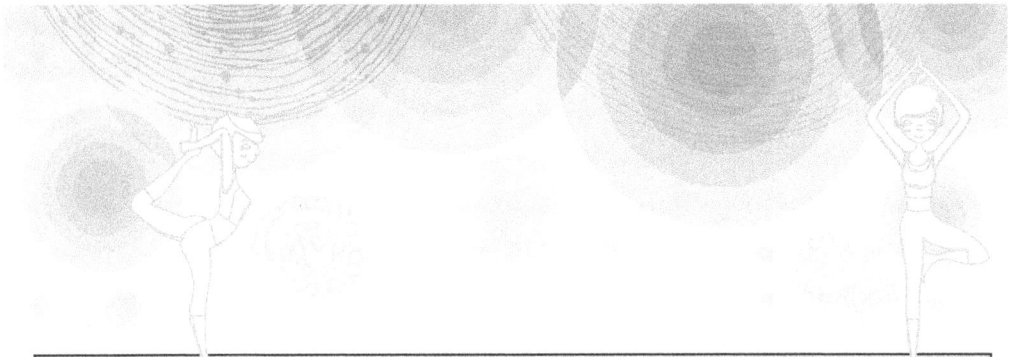

FOOD LOG

BREAKFAST	NOTES

SNACK	NOTES

LUNCH	NOTES

SNACK	NOTES

DINNER	NOTES

NUTRIENT TRACKER

	# OF SERVINGS						
GRAIN							
VEGGIES							
FRUITS							
DAIRY							
PROTEIN							
FATS							
VITAMINS							
SUGAR							

NOTES

HOURS OF SLEEP: _____
GLASSES OF WATER FOR TODAY : _____

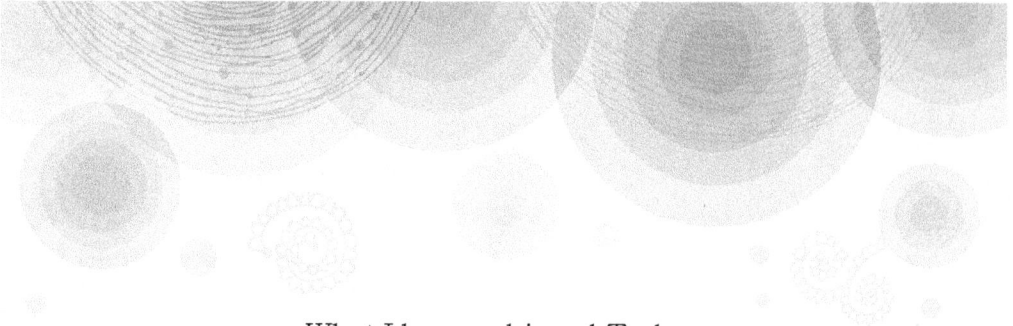

What I have achieved Today

_____

_____

_____

_____

_____

_____

What I need to improve next

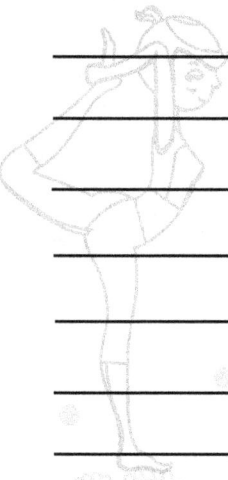

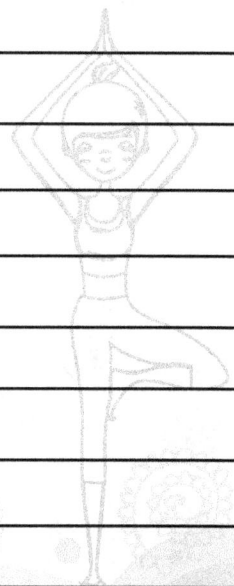

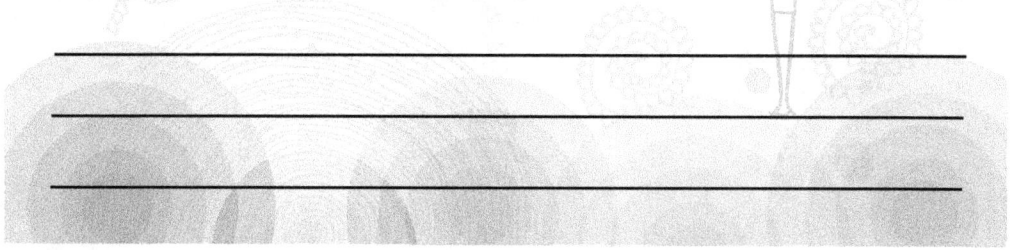

_____

_____

_____

_____

_____

_____

_____

_____

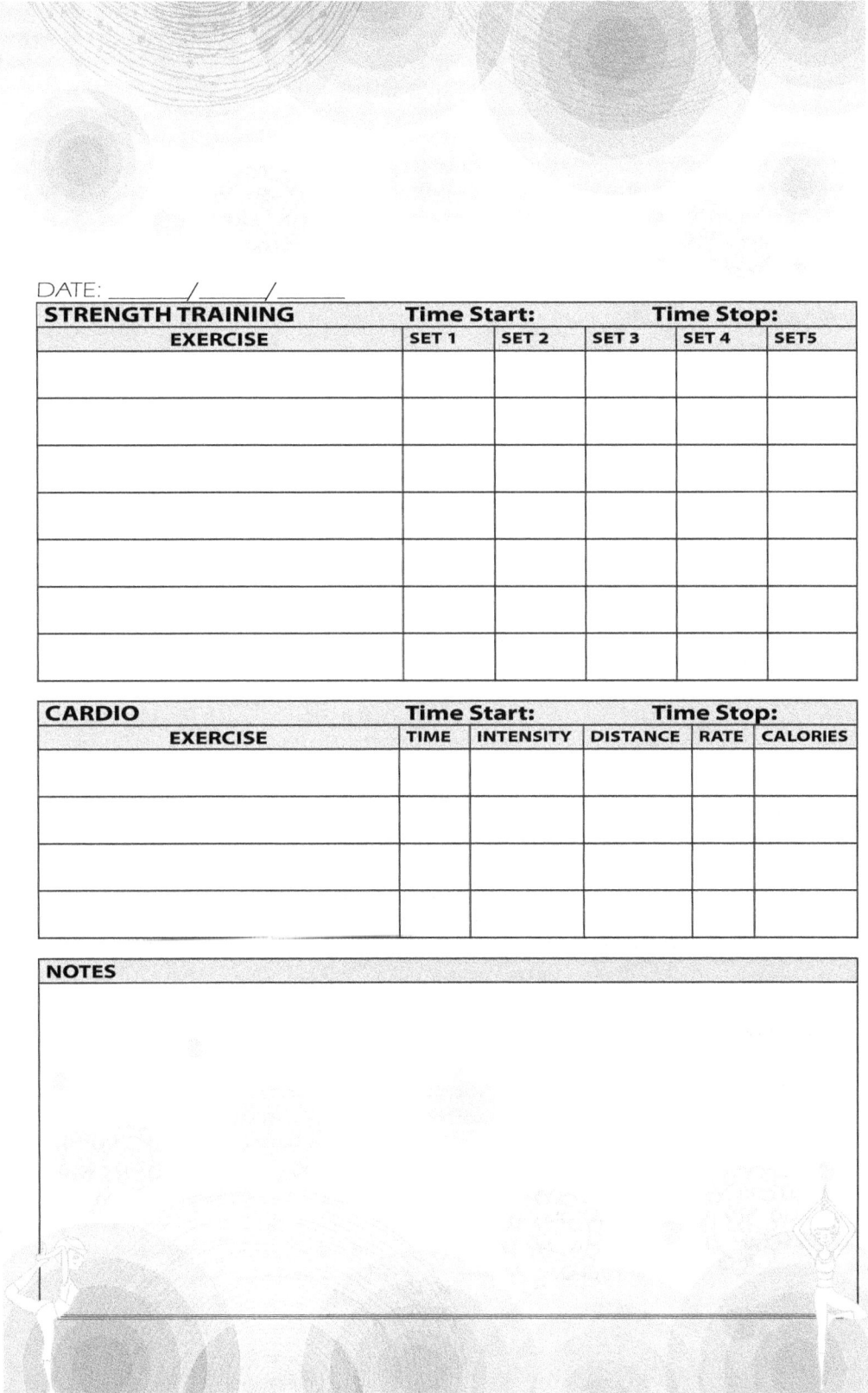

DATE: _____/_____/_____

STRENGTH TRAINING Time Start: Time Stop:

EXERCISE	SET 1	SET 2	SET 3	SET 4	SET5

CARDIO Time Start: Time Stop:

EXERCISE	TIME	INTENSITY	DISTANCE	RATE	CALORIES

NOTES

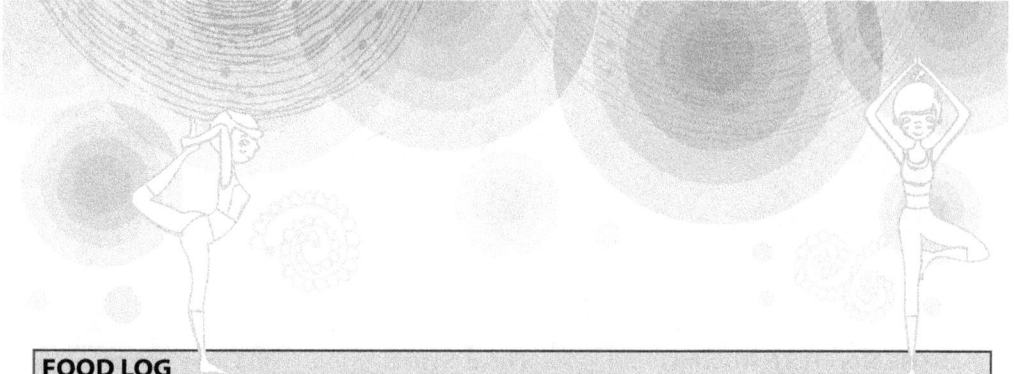

FOOD LOG

BREAKFAST	NOTES

SNACK	NOTES

LUNCH	NOTES

SNACK	NOTES

DINNER	NOTES

NUTRIENT TRACKER

	# OF SERVINGS					
GRAIN						
VEGGIES						
FRUITS						
DAIRY						
PROTEIN						
FATS						
VITAMINS						
SUGAR						

NOTES

HOURS OF SLEEP: _____

GLASSES OF WATER FOR TODAY : _____

What I have achieved Today

_____

_____

_____

_____

_____

What I need to improve next

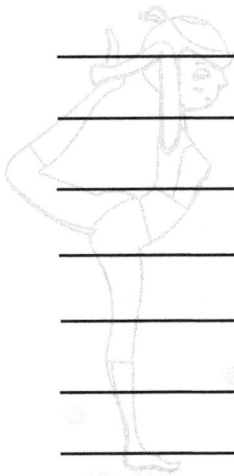

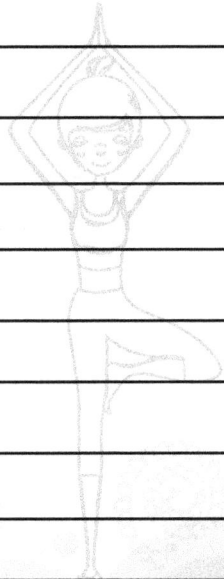

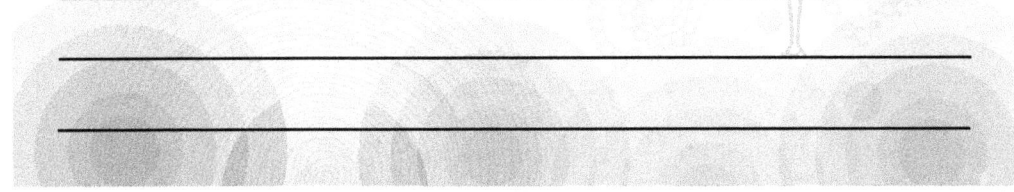

_____

_____

_____

_____

_____

_____

_____

_____

_____

_____

DATE: _____/_____/_____

STRENGTH TRAINING	Time Start:		Time Stop:		
EXERCISE	SET 1	SET 2	SET 3	SET 4	SET5

CARDIO	Time Start:		Time Stop:		
EXERCISE	TIME	INTENSITY	DISTANCE	RATE	CALORIES

NOTES

FOOD LOG

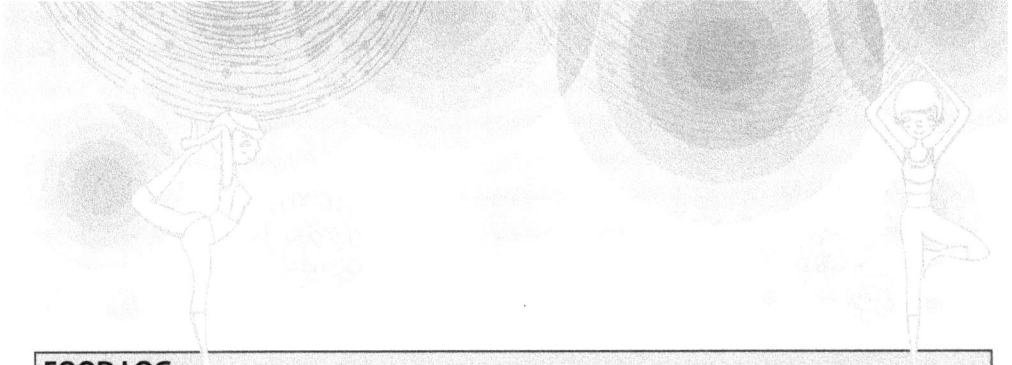

BREAKFAST	NOTES
SNACK	NOTES
LUNCH	NOTES
SNACK	NOTES
DINNER	NOTES

NUTRIENT TRACKER

	# OF SERVINGS						
GRAIN							
VEGGIES							
FRUITS							
DAIRY							
PROTEIN							
FATS							
VITAMINS							
SUGAR							

NOTES

HOURS OF SLEEP: _____
GLASSES OF WATER FOR TODAY : _____

What I have achieved Today

_____

_____

_____

_____

_____

What I need to improve next

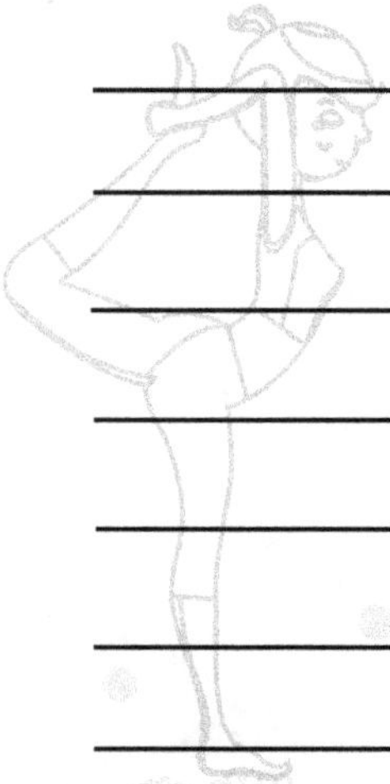

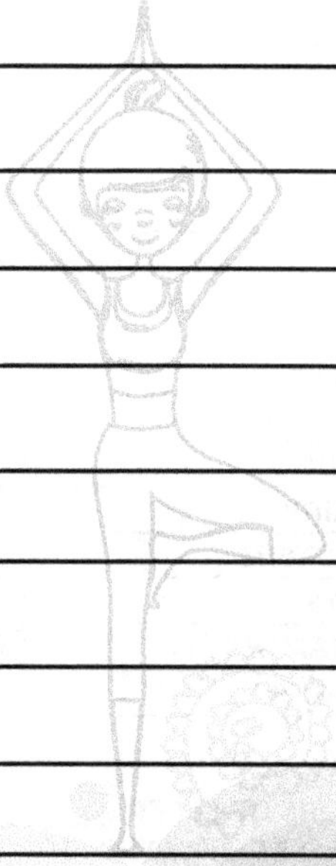

_____

_____

_____

_____

_____

_____

_____

_____

_____

DATE: _____ / _____ / _____

STRENGTH TRAINING   Time Start: Time Stop:

EXERCISE	SET 1	SET 2	SET 3	SET 4	SET5

CARDIO   Time Start: Time Stop:

EXERCISE	TIME	INTENSITY	DISTANCE	RATE	CALORIES

NOTES

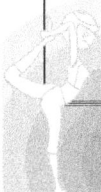
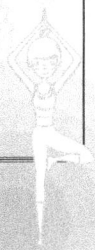

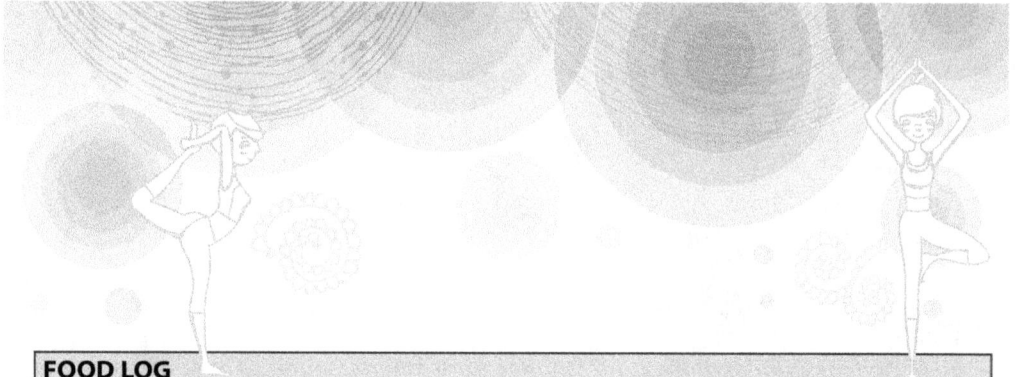

FOOD LOG

BREAKFAST	NOTES

SNACK	NOTES

LUNCH	NOTES

SNACK	NOTES

DINNER	NOTES

NUTRIENT TRACKER

	# OF SERVINGS						
GRAIN							
VEGGIES							
FRUITS							
DAIRY							
PROTEIN							
FATS							
VITAMINS							
SUGAR							

NOTES

HOURS OF SLEEP: _____
GLASSES OF WATER FOR TODAY : _____

What I have achieved Today

_____

_____

_____

_____

_____

_____

What I need to improve next

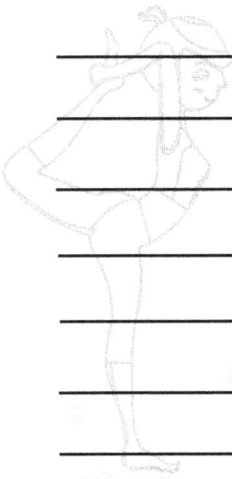

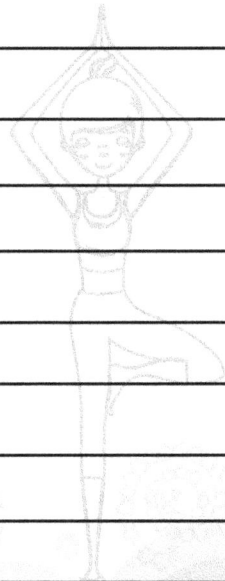

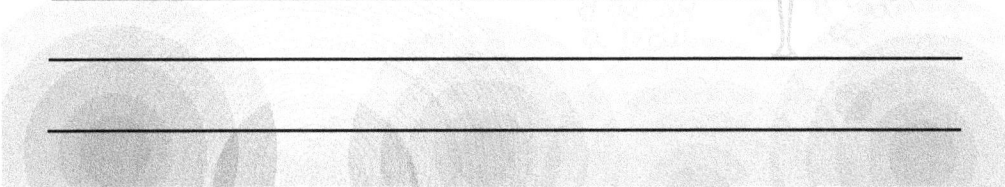

_____

_____

_____

_____

_____

_____

_____

_____

_____

_____

DATE: _____ / _____ / _____

STRENGTH TRAINING	Time Start:		Time Stop:		
EXERCISE	SET 1	SET 2	SET 3	SET 4	SET5

CARDIO	Time Start:		Time Stop:		
EXERCISE	TIME	INTENSITY	DISTANCE	RATE	CALORIES

NOTES

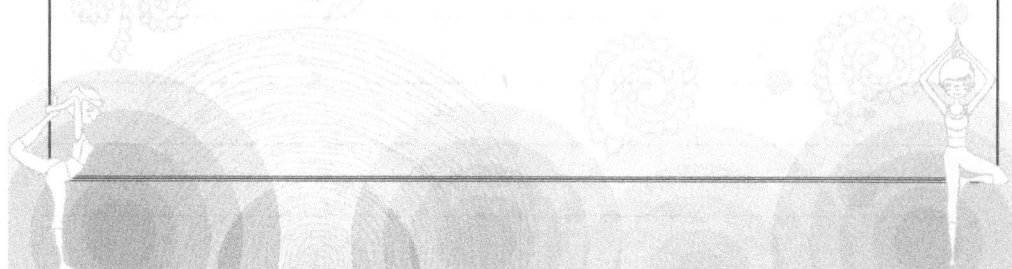

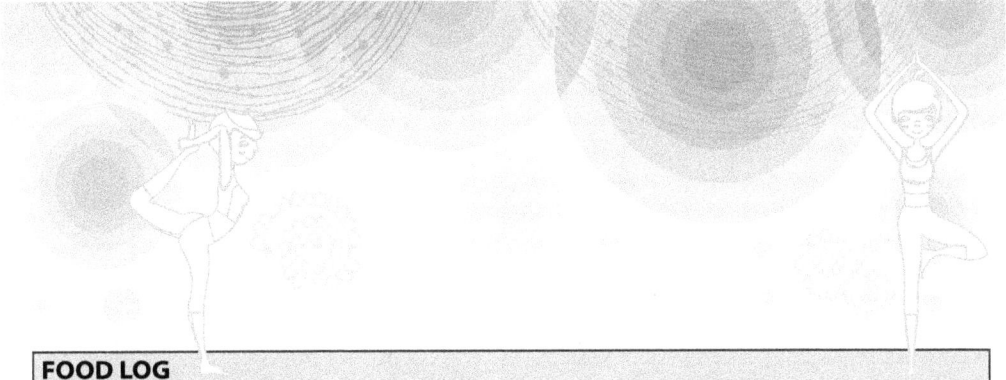

FOOD LOG

BREAKFAST	NOTES

SNACK	NOTES

LUNCH	NOTES

SNACK	NOTES

DINNER	NOTES

NUTRIENT TRACKER

	# OF SERVINGS						
GRAIN							
VEGGIES							
FRUITS							
DAIRY							
PROTEIN							
FATS							
VITAMINS							
SUGAR							

HOURS OF SLEEP: _____
GLASSES OF WATER FOR TODAY : _____

NOTES

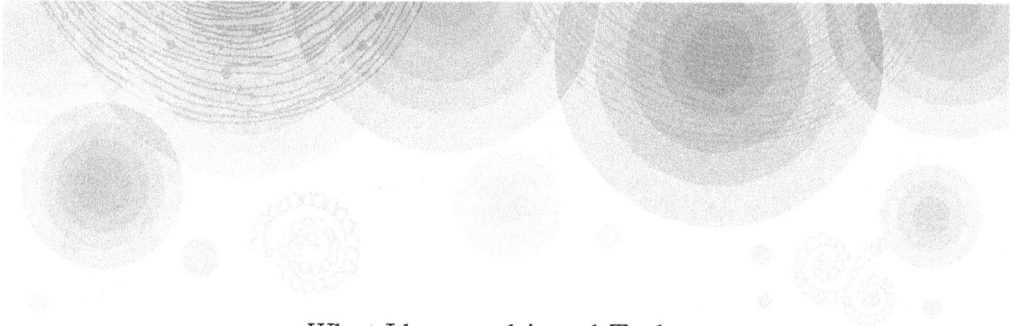

What I have achieved Today

_____

_____

_____

_____

_____

What I need to improve next

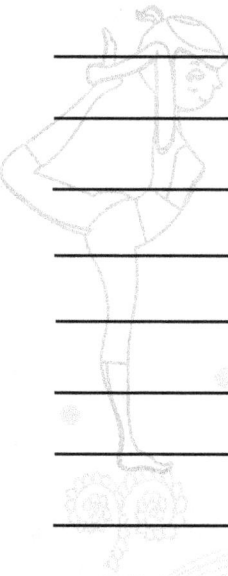

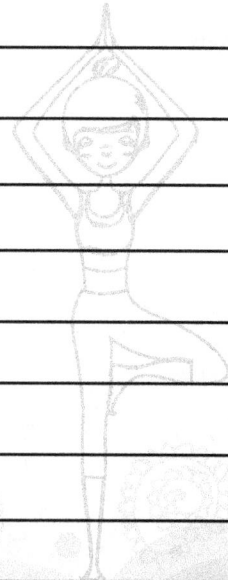

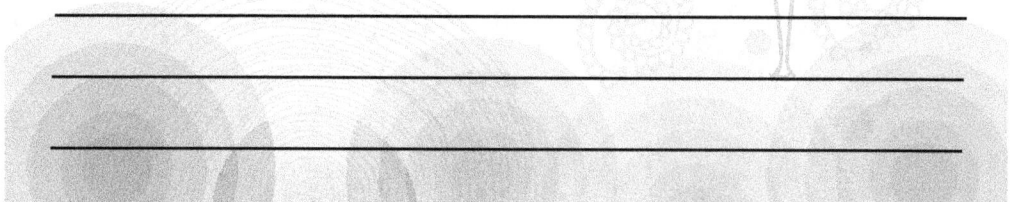

_____

_____

_____

_____

_____

_____

_____

_____

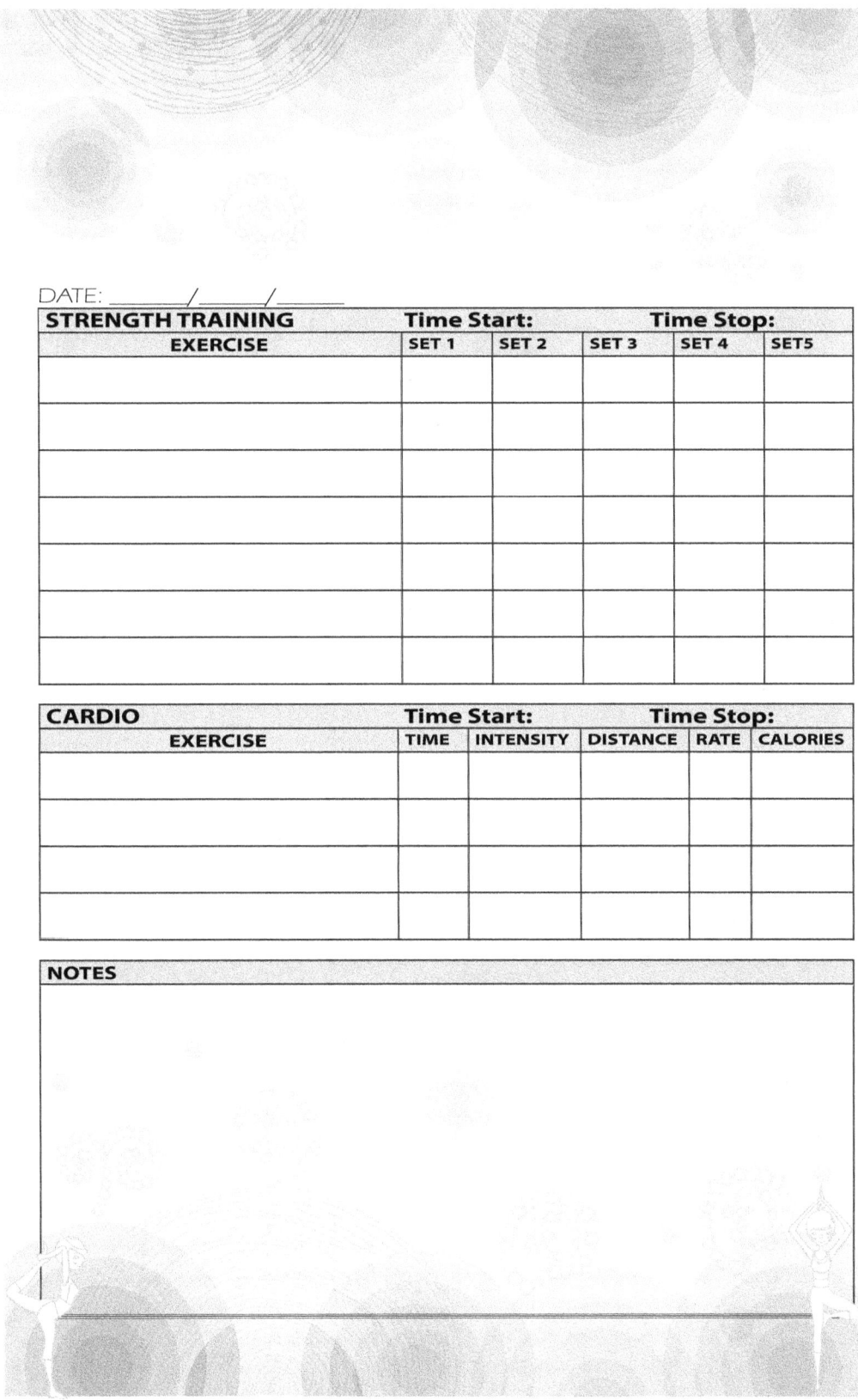

DATE: _____/_____/_____

STRENGTH TRAINING	Time Start:		Time Stop:		
EXERCISE	SET 1	SET 2	SET 3	SET 4	SET5

CARDIO	Time Start:		Time Stop:		
EXERCISE	TIME	INTENSITY	DISTANCE	RATE	CALORIES

NOTES

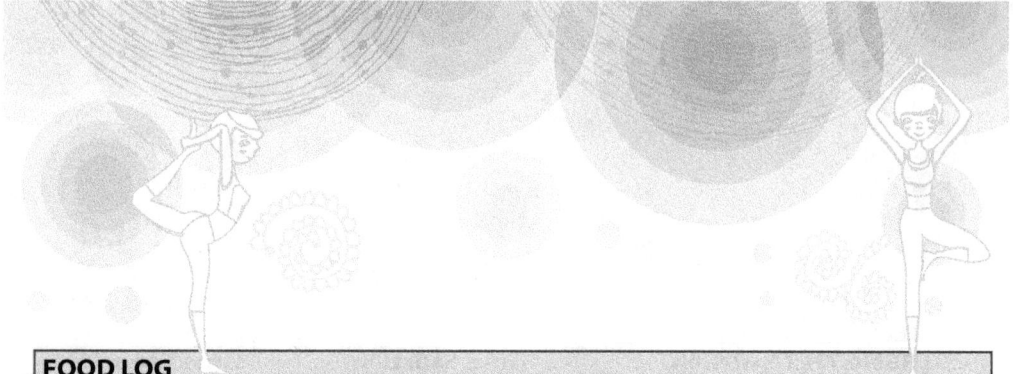

FOOD LOG	
BREAKFAST	**NOTES**
SNACK	**NOTES**
LUNCH	**NOTES**
SNACK	**NOTES**
DINNER	**NOTES**

NUTRIENT TRACKER

	# OF SERVINGS						
GRAIN							
VEGGIES							
FRUITS							
DAIRY							
PROTEIN							
FATS							
VITAMINS							
SUGAR							

NOTES

HOURS OF SLEEP: _____

GLASSES OF WATER FOR TODAY : _____

What I have achieved Today

_____

_____

_____

_____

_____

What I need to improve next

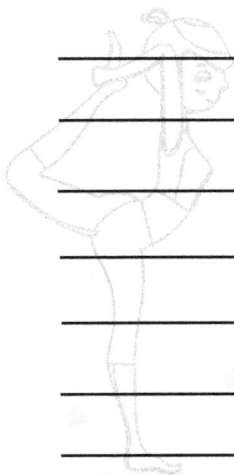

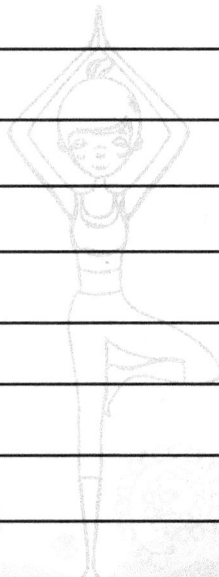

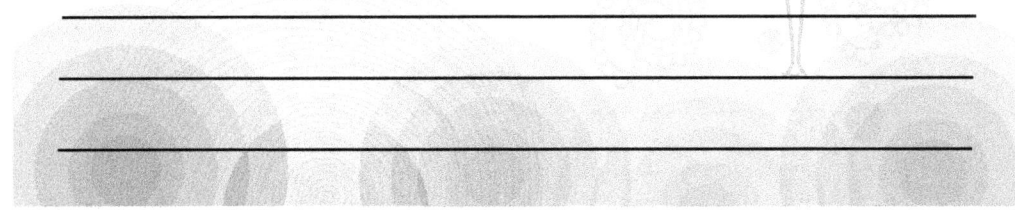

_____

_____

_____

_____

_____

_____

_____

_____

_____

_____

DATE: _____/_____/_____

STRENGTH TRAINING		Time Start:		Time Stop:		
EXERCISE	SET 1	SET 2	SET 3	SET 4	SET5

CARDIO		Time Start:		Time Stop:		
EXERCISE	TIME	INTENSITY	DISTANCE	RATE	CALORIES

NOTES

FOOD LOG

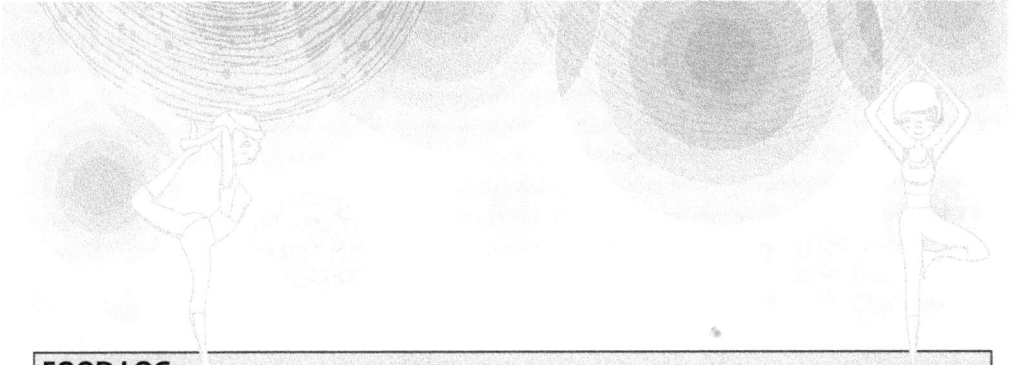

BREAKFAST	NOTES
SNACK	**NOTES**
LUNCH	**NOTES**
SNACK	**NOTES**
DINNER	**NOTES**

NUTRIENT TRACKER

	# OF SERVINGS						
GRAIN							
VEGGIES							
FRUITS							
DAIRY							
PROTEIN							
FATS							
VITAMINS							
SUGAR							

NOTES

HOURS OF SLEEP: _____
GLASSES OF WATER FOR TODAY : _____

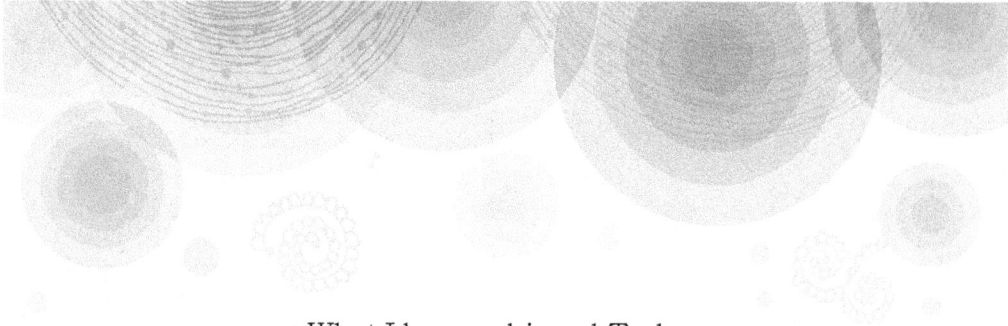

What I have achieved Today

_____

_____

_____

_____

_____

What I need to improve next

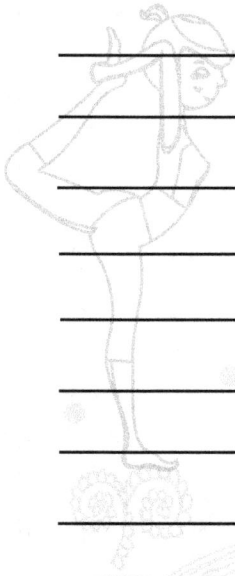

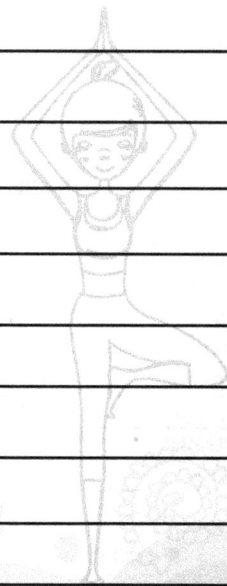

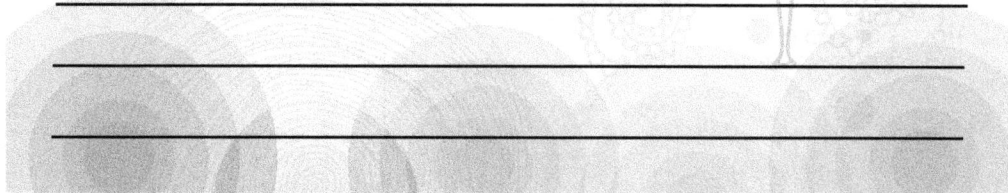

_____

_____

_____

_____

_____

_____

_____

_____

_____

DATE: _____ / _____ / _____

STRENGTH TRAINING   Time Start: Time Stop:

EXERCISE	SET 1	SET 2	SET 3	SET 4	SET5

CARDIO   Time Start: Time Stop:

EXERCISE	TIME	INTENSITY	DISTANCE	RATE	CALORIES

NOTES

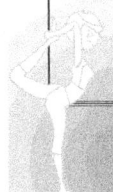

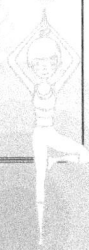

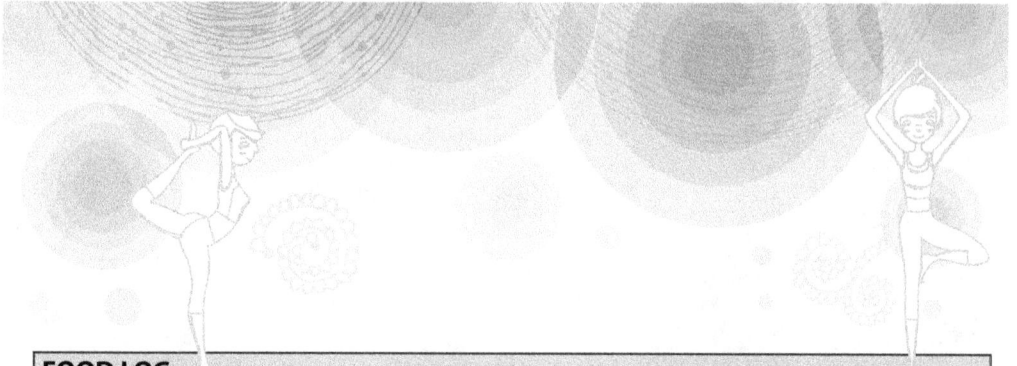

FOOD LOG

BREAKFAST	NOTES

SNACK	NOTES

LUNCH	NOTES

SNACK	NOTES

DINNER	NOTES

NUTRIENT TRACKER

	# OF SERVINGS							
GRAIN								
VEGGIES								
FRUITS								
DAIRY								
PROTEIN								
FATS								
VITAMINS								
SUGAR								

NOTES

HOURS OF SLEEP: _____
GLASSES OF WATER FOR TODAY : _____

What I have achieved Today

_____

_____

_____

_____

_____

_____

What I need to improve next

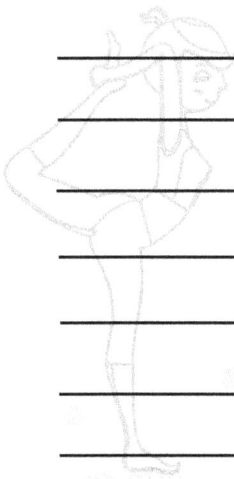

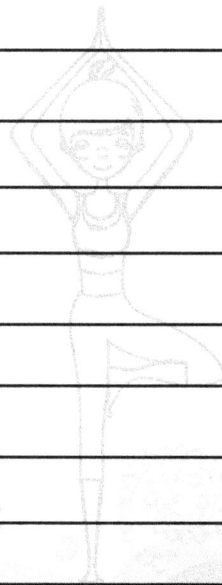

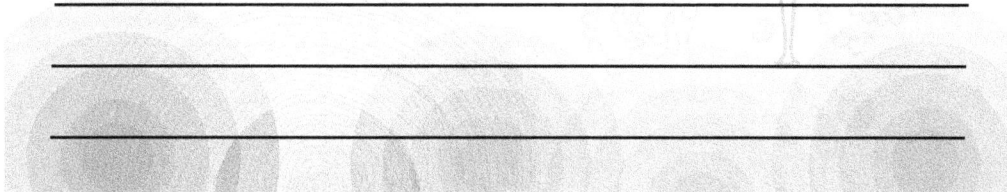

_____

_____

_____

_____

_____

_____

_____

_____

_____

_____

DATE: _____/_____/_____

STRENGTH TRAINING		Time Start:			Time Stop:	
EXERCISE	SET 1	SET 2	SET 3	SET 4	SET5

CARDIO		Time Start:			Time Stop:	
EXERCISE	TIME	INTENSITY	DISTANCE	RATE	CALORIES

NOTES

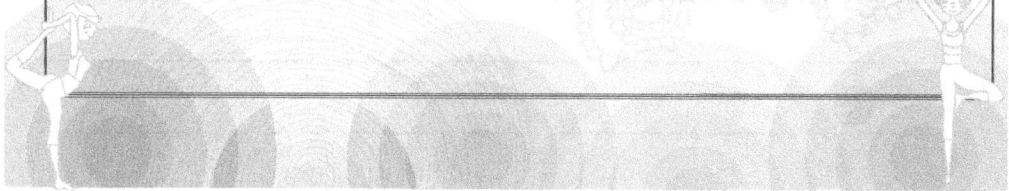

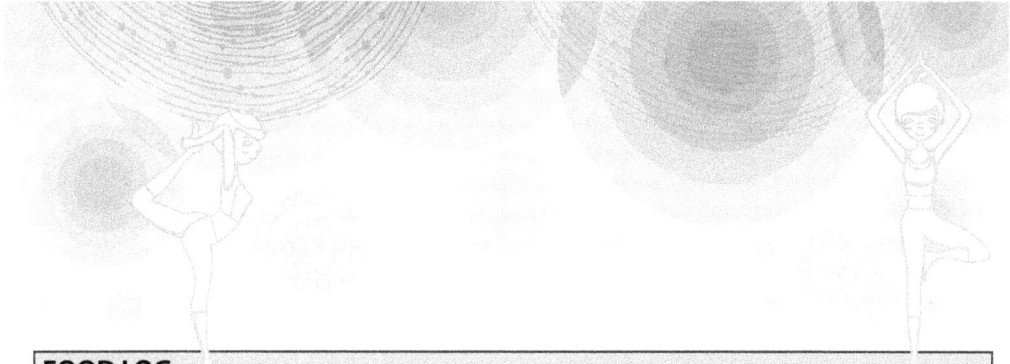

FOOD LOG

BREAKFAST	NOTES

SNACK	NOTES

LUNCH	NOTES

SNACK	NOTES

DINNER	NOTES

NUTRIENT TRACKER

	# OF SERVINGS						
GRAIN							
VEGGIES							
FRUITS							
DAIRY							
PROTEIN							
FATS							
VITAMINS							
SUGAR							

NOTES

HOURS OF SLEEP: _____
GLASSES OF WATER FOR TODAY : _____

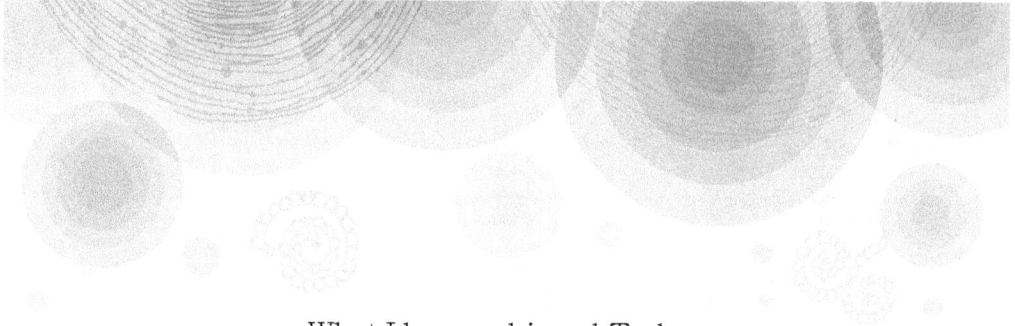

What I have achieved Today

_____

_____

_____

_____

_____

_____

What I need to improve next

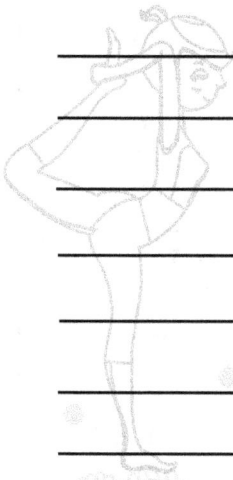

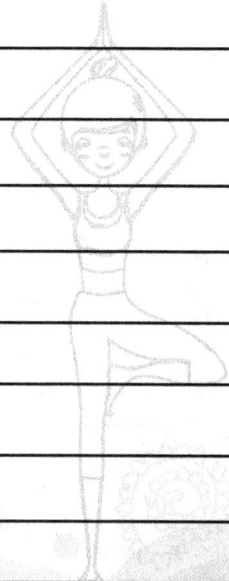

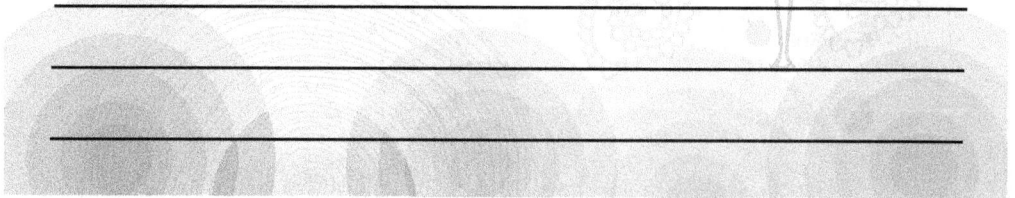

_____

_____

_____

_____

_____

_____

_____

_____

_____

DATE: _____ / _____ / _____

STRENGTH TRAINING	Time Start:		Time Stop:		
EXERCISE	SET 1	SET 2	SET 3	SET 4	SET5

CARDIO	Time Start:		Time Stop:		
EXERCISE	TIME	INTENSITY	DISTANCE	RATE	CALORIES

NOTES

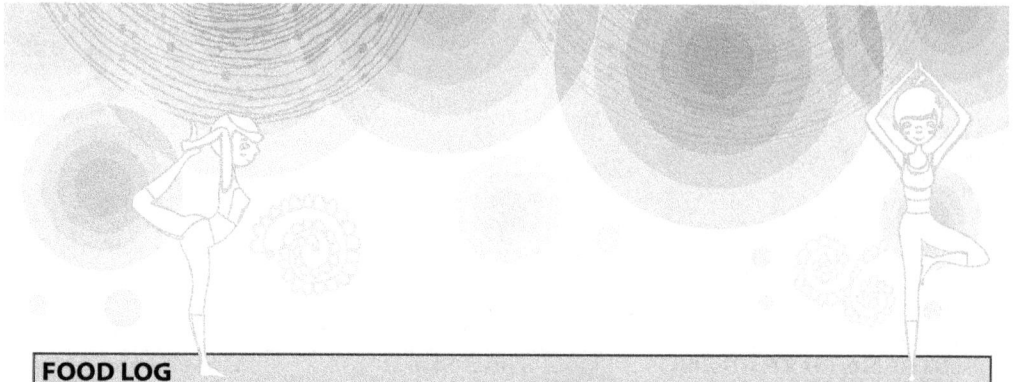

FOOD LOG

BREAKFAST	NOTES

SNACK	NOTES

LUNCH	NOTES

SNACK	NOTES

DINNER	NOTES

NUTRIENT TRACKER

	# OF SERVINGS						
GRAIN							
VEGGIES							
FRUITS							
DAIRY							
PROTEIN							
FATS							
VITAMINS							
SUGAR							

NOTES

HOURS OF SLEEP: _____
GLASSES OF WATER FOR TODAY : _____

What I have achieved Today

_____

_____

_____

_____

_____

What I need to improve next

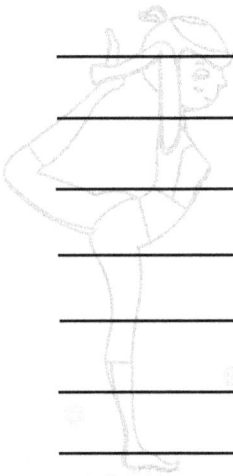

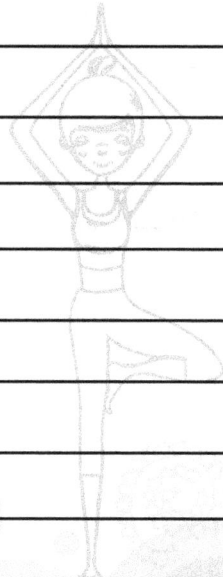

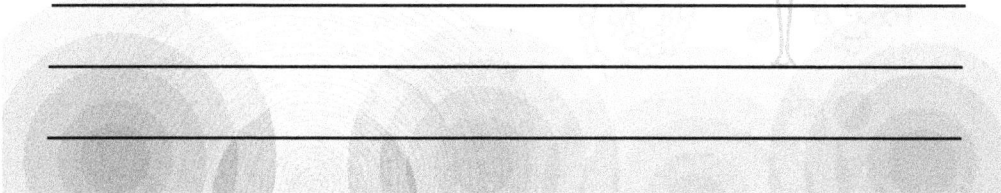

_____

_____

_____

_____

_____

_____

_____

_____

_____

_____

DATE: _____/_____/_____

STRENGTH TRAINING	Time Start:		Time Stop:		
EXERCISE	**SET 1**	**SET 2**	**SET 3**	**SET 4**	**SET5**

CARDIO	Time Start:		Time Stop:		
EXERCISE	**TIME**	**INTENSITY**	**DISTANCE**	**RATE**	**CALORIES**

NOTES

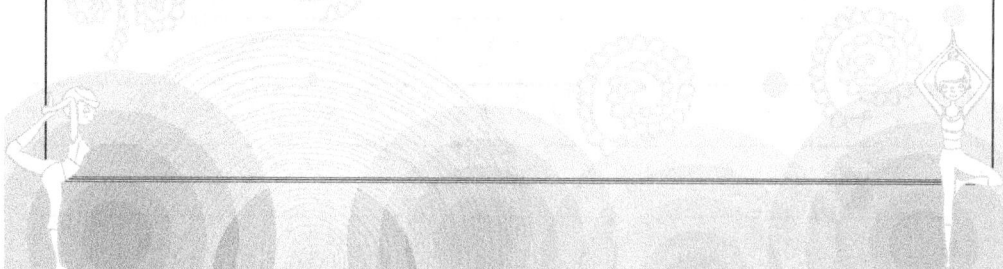

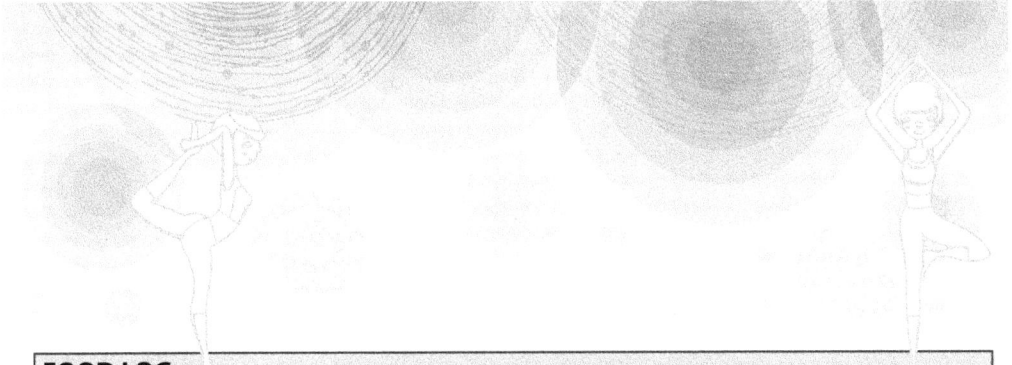

FOOD LOG

BREAKFAST	NOTES

SNACK	NOTES

LUNCH	NOTES

SNACK	NOTES

DINNER	NOTES

NUTRIENT TRACKER

	# OF SERVINGS							
GRAIN								
VEGGIES								
FRUITS								
DAIRY								
PROTEIN								
FATS								
VITAMINS								
SUGAR								

HOURS OF SLEEP: _____
GLASSES OF WATER FOR TODAY : _____

NOTES

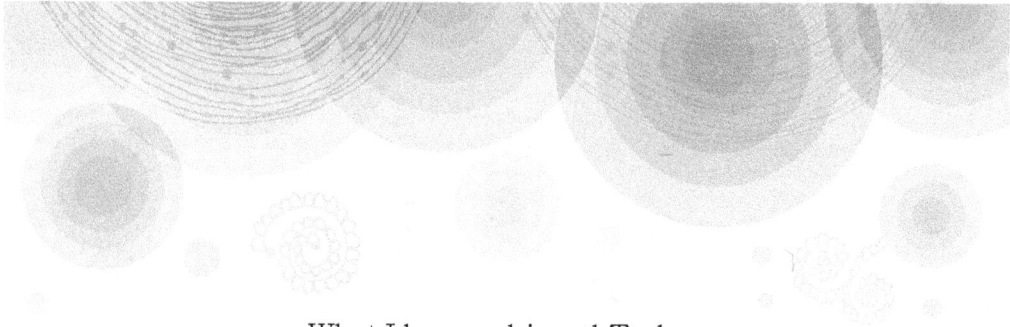

What I have achieved Today

_____

_____

_____

_____

_____

What I need to improve next

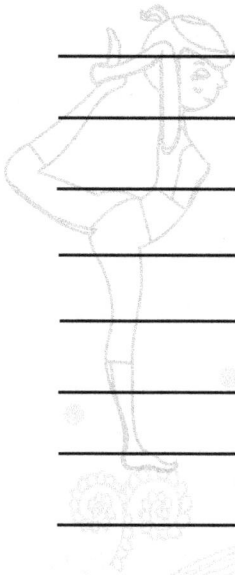

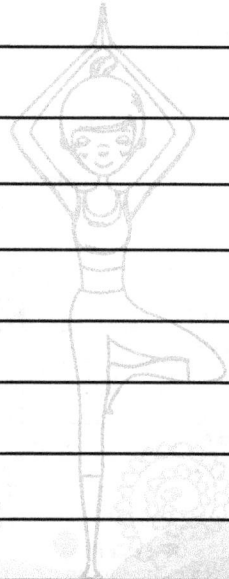

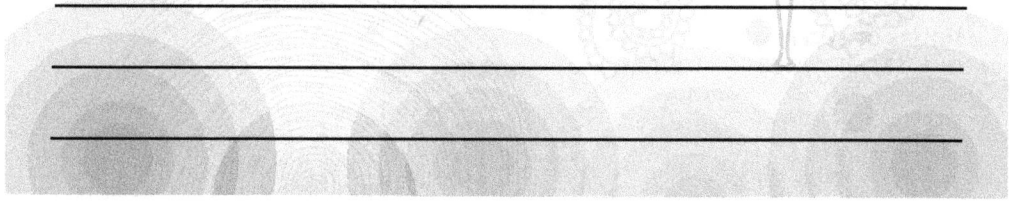

_____

_____

_____

_____

_____

_____

_____

_____

_____

DATE: _____/_____/_____

STRENGTH TRAINING	Time Start:		Time Stop:		
EXERCISE	SET 1	SET 2	SET 3	SET 4	SET5

CARDIO	Time Start:		Time Stop:		
EXERCISE	TIME	INTENSITY	DISTANCE	RATE	CALORIES

NOTES

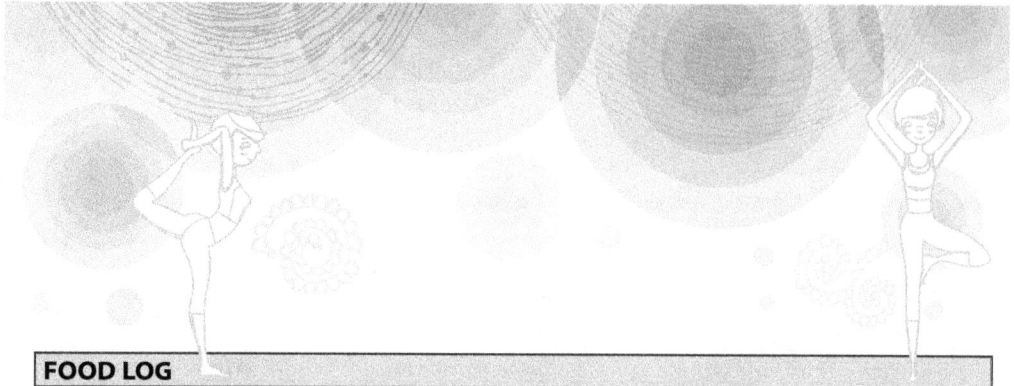

FOOD LOG

BREAKFAST	NOTES

SNACK	NOTES

LUNCH	NOTES

SNACK	NOTES

DINNER	NOTES

NUTRIENT TRACKER

	# OF SERVINGS						
GRAIN							
VEGGIES							
FRUITS							
DAIRY							
PROTEIN							
FATS							
VITAMINS							
SUGAR							

HOURS OF SLEEP: _____

GLASSES OF WATER FOR TODAY : _____

NOTES

What I have achieved Today

_____

_____

_____

_____

_____

_____

What I need to improve next

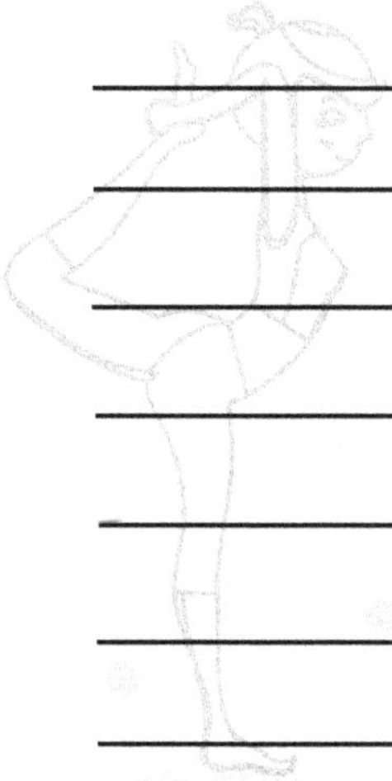

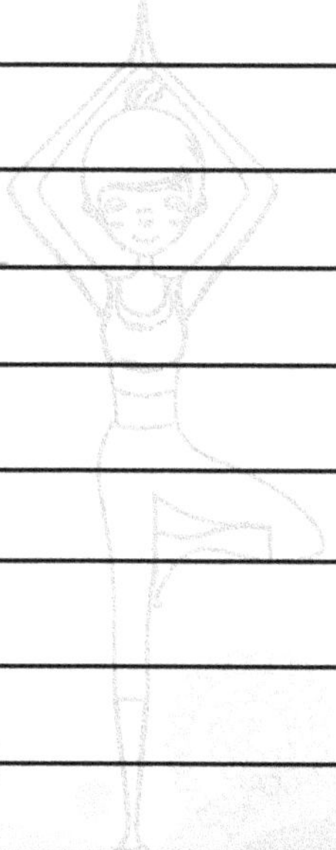

_____

_____

_____

_____

_____

_____

_____

_____

_____

_____

DATE: _____/_____/_____

STRENGTH TRAINING   Time Start: Time Stop:

EXERCISE	SET 1	SET 2	SET 3	SET 4	SET5

CARDIO   Time Start: Time Stop:

EXERCISE	TIME	INTENSITY	DISTANCE	RATE	CALORIES

NOTES

FOOD LOG

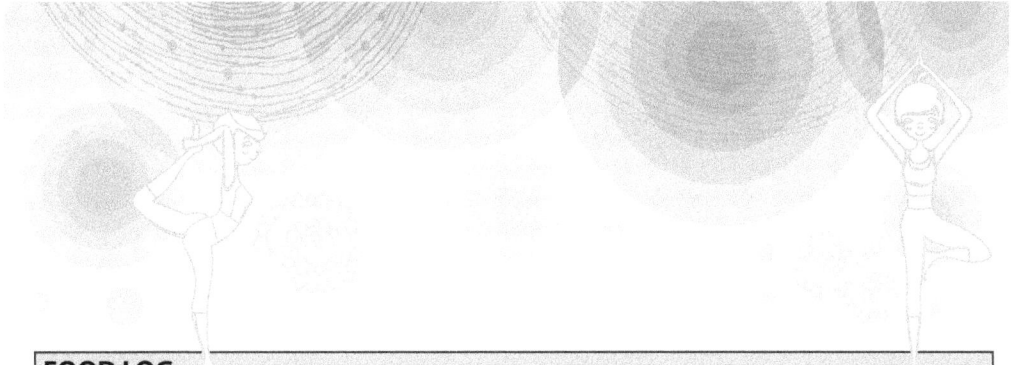

BREAKFAST	NOTES
SNACK	NOTES
LUNCH	NOTES
SNACK	NOTES
DINNER	NOTES

NUTRIENT TRACKER

	# OF SERVINGS						
GRAIN							
VEGGIES							
FRUITS							
DAIRY							
PROTEIN							
FATS							
VITAMINS							
SUGAR							

NOTES

HOURS OF SLEEP: _____

GLASSES OF WATER FOR TODAY : _____

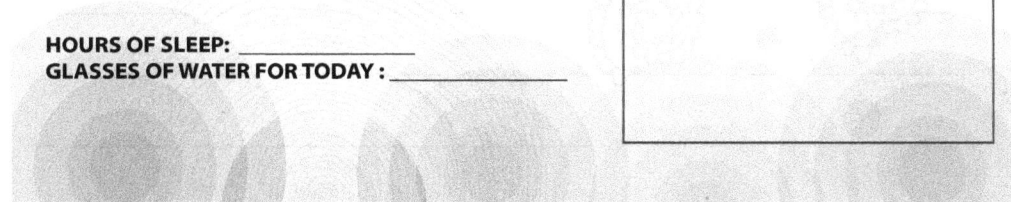

What I have achieved Today

_____

_____

_____

_____

_____

What I need to improve next

_____

_____

_____

_____

_____

_____

_____

_____

_____

DATE: _____/_____/_____

STRENGTH TRAINING		Time Start:			Time Stop:	
EXERCISE	SET 1	SET 2	SET 3	SET 4	SET5

CARDIO		Time Start:		Time Stop:		
EXERCISE	TIME	INTENSITY	DISTANCE	RATE	CALORIES

NOTES

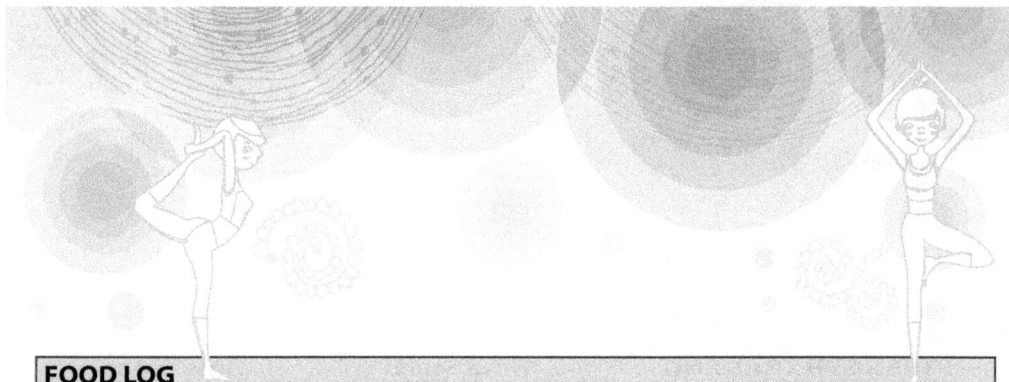

FOOD LOG

BREAKFAST	NOTES

SNACK	NOTES

LUNCH	NOTES

SNACK	NOTES

DINNER	NOTES

NUTRIENT TRACKER

	# OF SERVINGS						
GRAIN							
VEGGIES							
FRUITS							
DAIRY							
PROTEIN							
FATS							
VITAMINS							
SUGAR							

NOTES

HOURS OF SLEEP: _____

GLASSES OF WATER FOR TODAY : _____

What I have achieved Today

_____

_____

_____

_____

_____

What I need to improve next

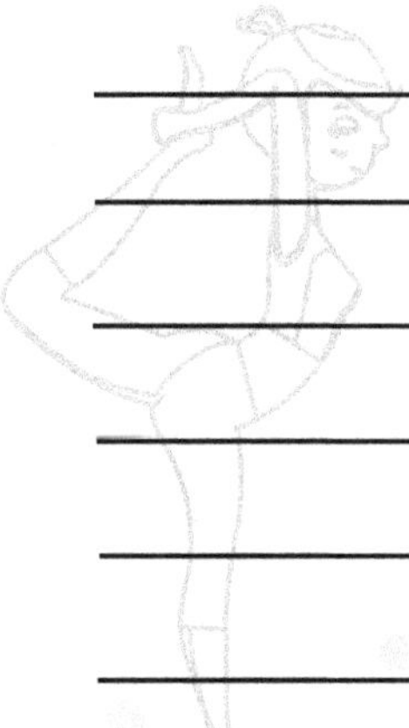

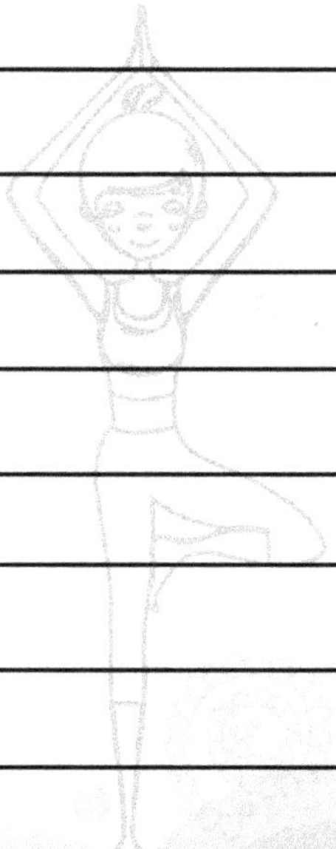

_____

_____

_____

_____

_____

_____

_____

_____

_____

_____

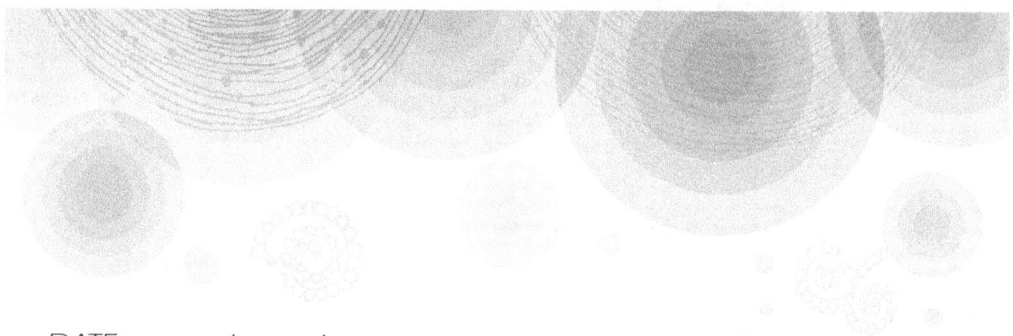

DATE: _____/_____/_____

STRENGTH TRAINING	Time Start:		Time Stop:		
EXERCISE	SET 1	SET 2	SET 3	SET 4	SET5

CARDIO	Time Start:		Time Stop:		
EXERCISE	TIME	INTENSITY	DISTANCE	RATE	CALORIES

NOTES

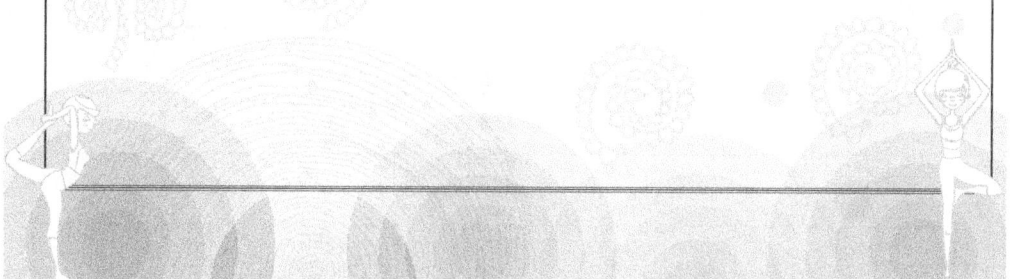

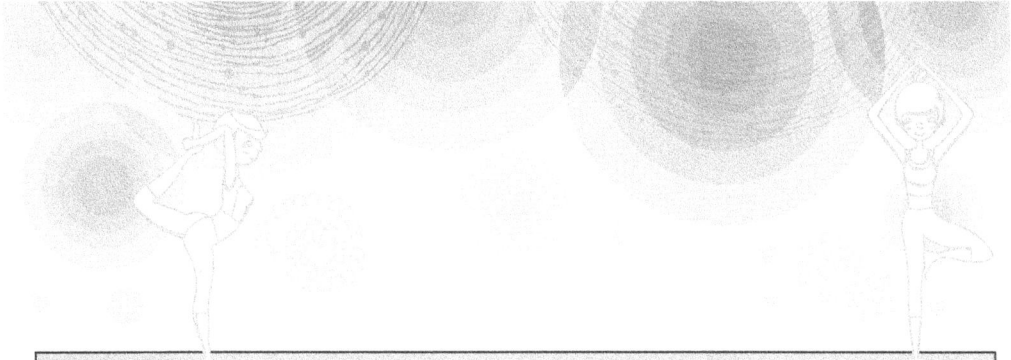

FOOD LOG

BREAKFAST	NOTES

SNACK	NOTES

LUNCH	NOTES

SNACK	NOTES

DINNER	NOTES

NUTRIENT TRACKER

	# OF SERVINGS						
GRAIN							
VEGGIES							
FRUITS							
DAIRY							
PROTEIN							
FATS							
VITAMINS							
SUGAR							

NOTES

HOURS OF SLEEP: _____
GLASSES OF WATER FOR TODAY : _____

What I have achieved Today

_____

_____

_____

_____

_____

What I need to improve next

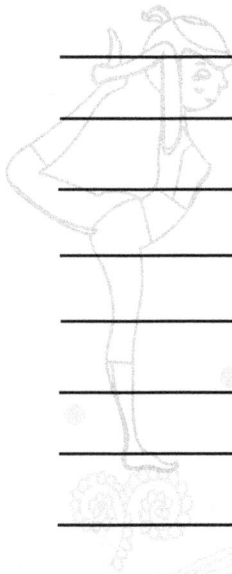

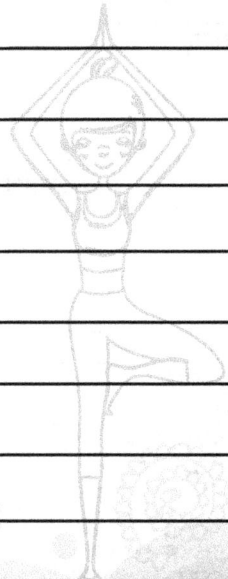

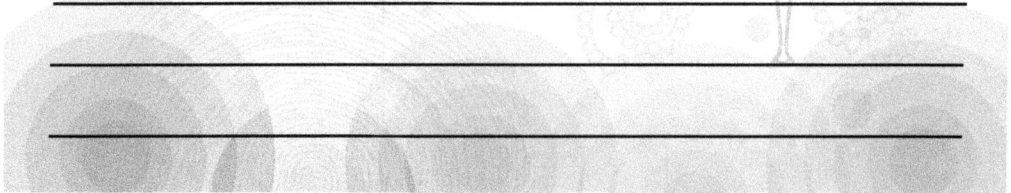

_____

_____

_____

_____

_____

_____

_____

_____

_____

DATE: _____ / _____ / _____

STRENGTH TRAINING		Time Start:		Time Stop:		
EXERCISE	SET 1	SET 2	SET 3	SET 4	SET5

CARDIO		Time Start:		Time Stop:		
EXERCISE	TIME	INTENSITY	DISTANCE	RATE	CALORIES

NOTES

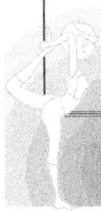
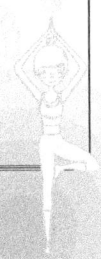

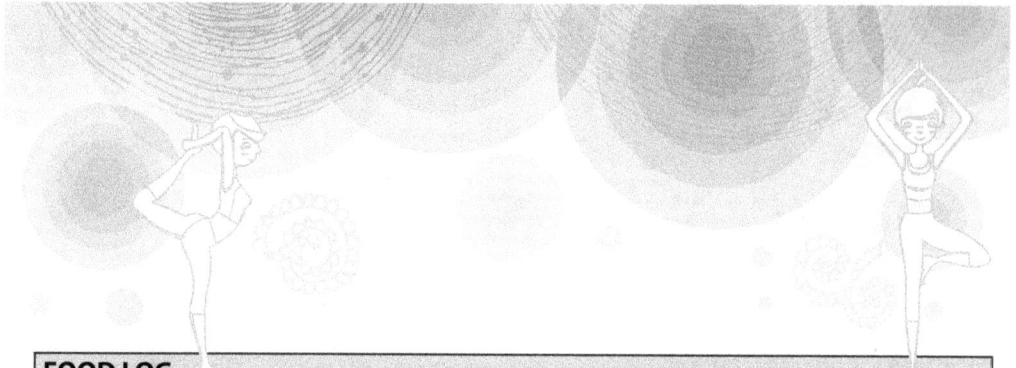

FOOD LOG

BREAKFAST	NOTES

SNACK	NOTES

LUNCH	NOTES

SNACK	NOTES

DINNER	NOTES

NUTRIENT TRACKER

	# OF SERVINGS						
GRAIN							
VEGGIES							
FRUITS							
DAIRY							
PROTEIN							
FATS							
VITAMINS							
SUGAR							

NOTES

HOURS OF SLEEP: _____

GLASSES OF WATER FOR TODAY : _____

What I have achieved Today

_____

_____

_____

_____

_____

What I need to improve next

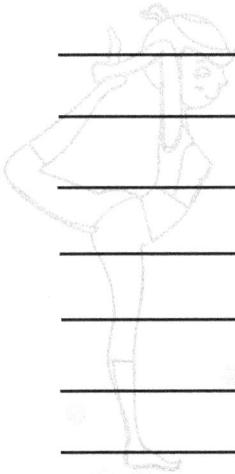

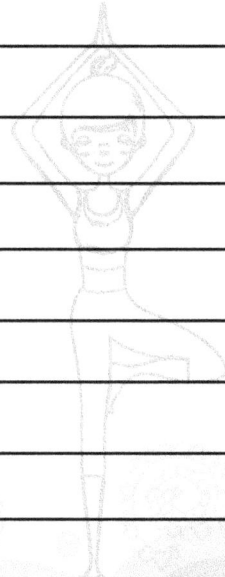

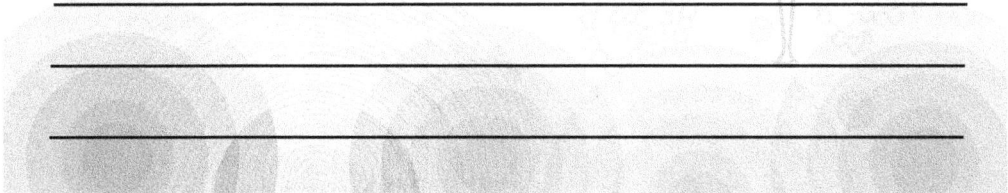

_____

_____

_____

_____

_____

_____

_____

_____

_____

_____

DATE: _____ / _____ / _____

STRENGTH TRAINING	Time Start:		Time Stop:		
EXERCISE	SET 1	SET 2	SET 3	SET 4	SET5

CARDIO	Time Start:		Time Stop:		
EXERCISE	TIME	INTENSITY	DISTANCE	RATE	CALORIES

NOTES

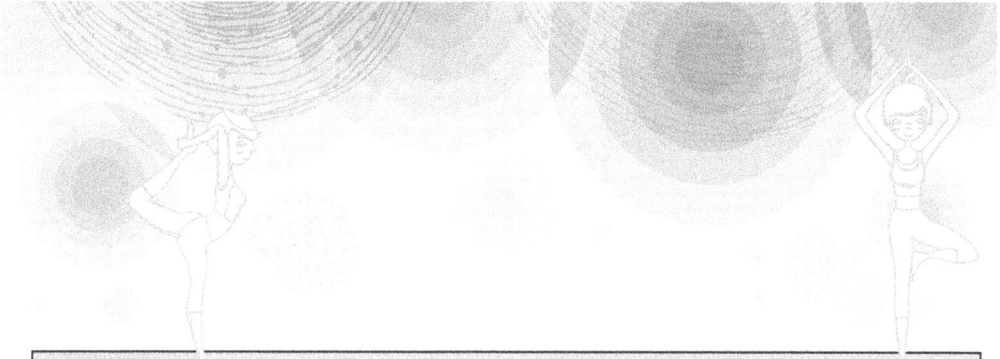

FOOD LOG

BREAKFAST	NOTES

SNACK	NOTES

LUNCH	NOTES

SNACK	NOTES

DINNER	NOTES

NUTRIENT TRACKER

	# OF SERVINGS						
GRAIN							
VEGGIES							
FRUITS							
DAIRY							
PROTEIN							
FATS							
VITAMINS							
SUGAR							

NOTES

HOURS OF SLEEP: _____
GLASSES OF WATER FOR TODAY : _____

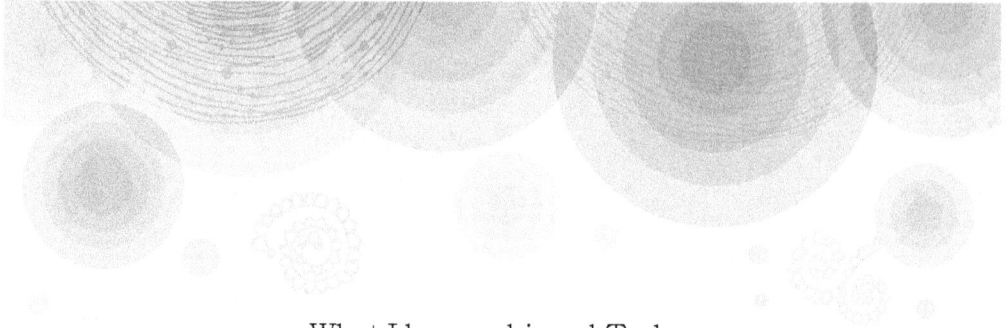

What I have achieved Today

_____

_____

_____

_____

_____

What I need to improve next

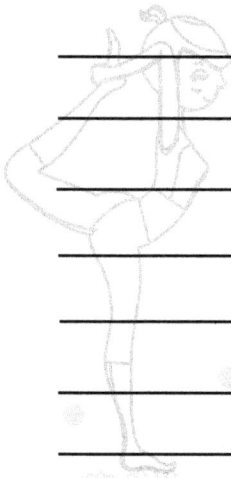

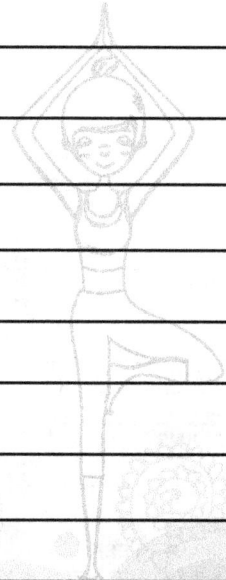

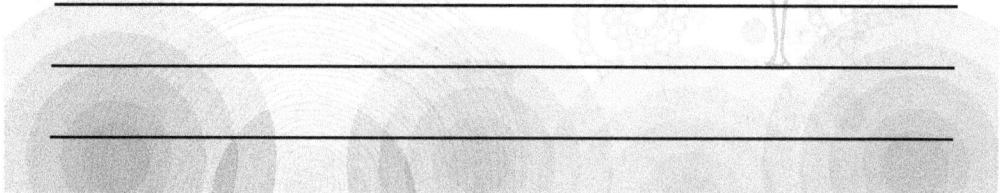

_____

_____

_____

_____

_____

_____

_____

_____

_____

DATE: _____ / _____ / _____

STRENGTH TRAINING	Time Start:			Time Stop:	
EXERCISE	SET 1	SET 2	SET 3	SET 4	SET5

CARDIO	Time Start:		Time Stop:		
EXERCISE	TIME	INTENSITY	DISTANCE	RATE	CALORIES

NOTES

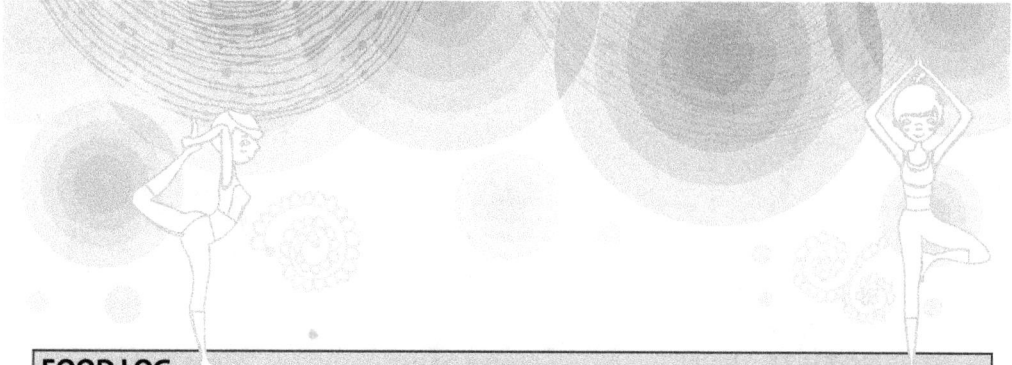

FOOD LOG

BREAKFAST	NOTES
SNACK	NOTES
LUNCH	NOTES
SNACK	NOTES
DINNER	NOTES

NUTRIENT TRACKER

	# OF SERVINGS						
GRAIN							
VEGGIES							
FRUITS							
DAIRY							
PROTEIN							
FATS							
VITAMINS							
SUGAR							

NOTES

HOURS OF SLEEP: _____

GLASSES OF WATER FOR TODAY : _____

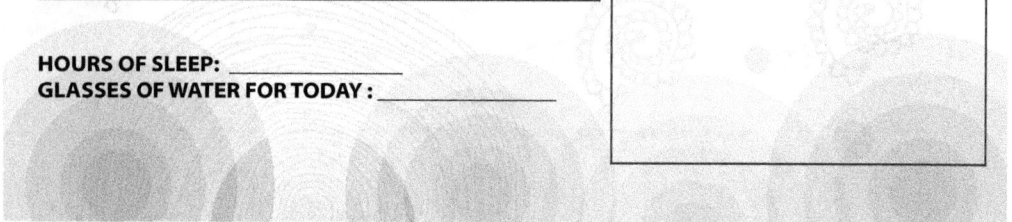

What I have achieved Today

_____

_____

_____

_____

_____

What I need to improve next

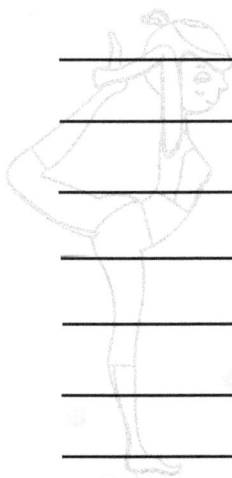

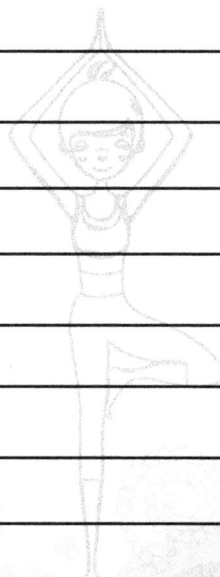

_____

_____

_____

_____

_____

_____

_____

_____

_____

_____

DATE: _____/_____/_____

STRENGTH TRAINING		Time Start:		Time Stop:		
EXERCISE	SET 1	SET 2	SET 3	SET 4	SET5

CARDIO		Time Start:		Time Stop:		
EXERCISE	TIME	INTENSITY	DISTANCE	RATE	CALORIES

NOTES

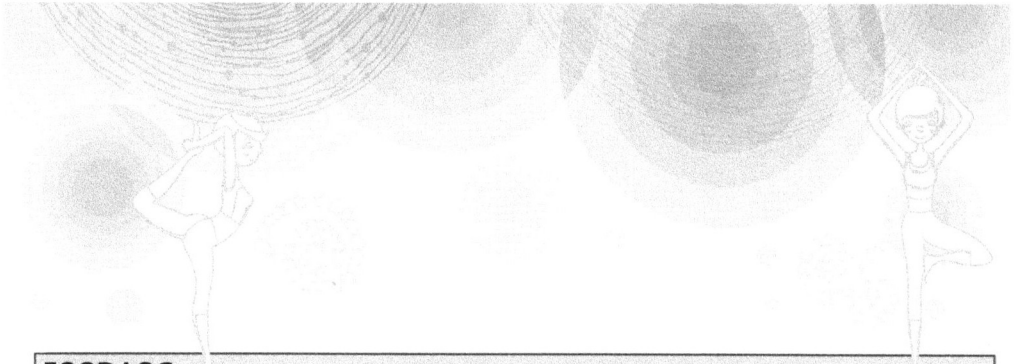

FOOD LOG

BREAKFAST	NOTES

SNACK	NOTES

LUNCH	NOTES

SNACK	NOTES

DINNER	NOTES

NUTRIENT TRACKER

	# OF SERVINGS						
GRAIN							
VEGGIES							
FRUITS							
DAIRY							
PROTEIN							
FATS							
VITAMINS							
SUGAR							

NOTES

HOURS OF SLEEP: _____

GLASSES OF WATER FOR TODAY : _____

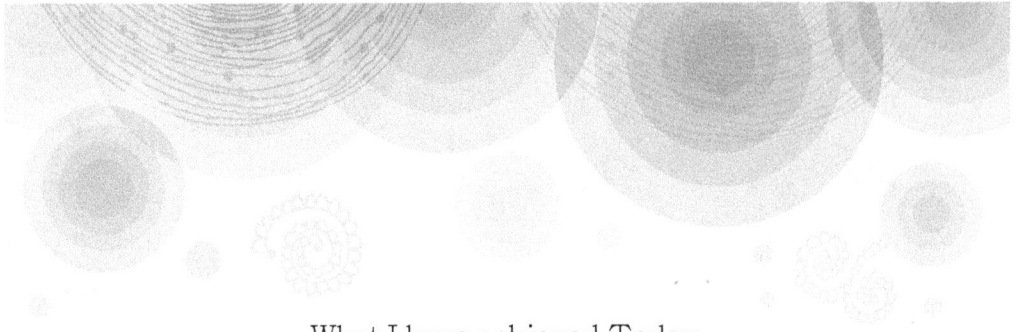

What I have achieved Today

_____

_____

_____

_____

_____

What I need to improve next

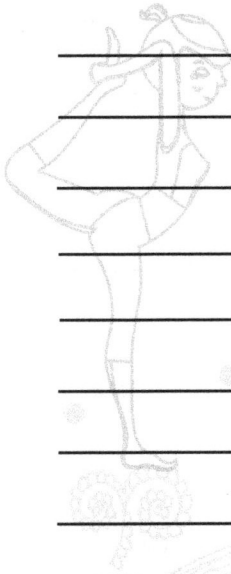

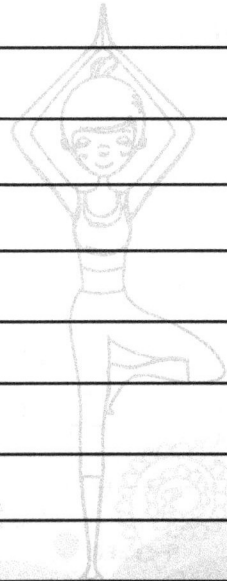

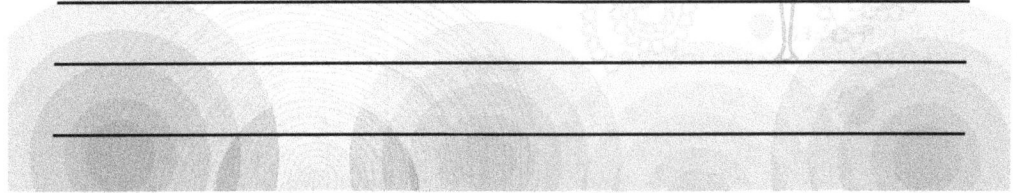

_____

_____

_____

_____

_____

_____

_____

_____

_____

DATE: _____ / _____ / _____

STRENGTH TRAINING	Time Start:		Time Stop:		
EXERCISE	SET 1	SET 2	SET 3	SET 4	SET5

CARDIO	Time Start:		Time Stop:		
EXERCISE	TIME	INTENSITY	DISTANCE	RATE	CALORIES

NOTES

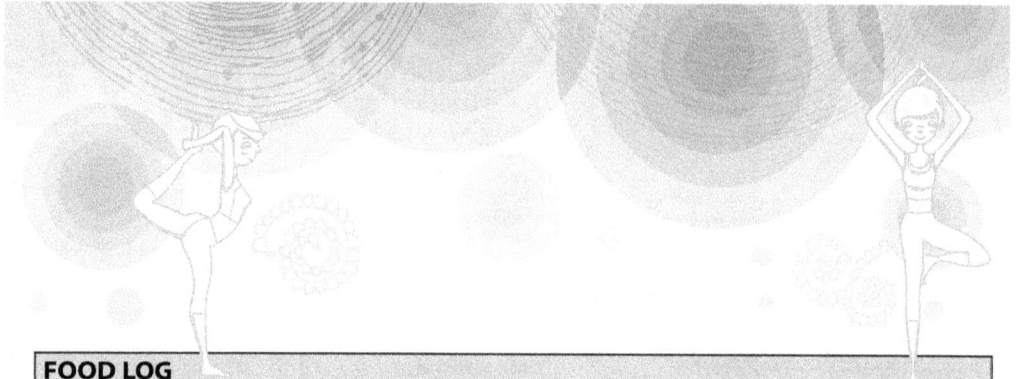

FOOD LOG

BREAKFAST	NOTES

SNACK	NOTES

LUNCH	NOTES

SNACK	NOTES

DINNER	NOTES

NUTRIENT TRACKER

	# OF SERVINGS						
GRAIN							
VEGGIES							
FRUITS							
DAIRY							
PROTEIN							
FATS							
VITAMINS							
SUGAR							

HOURS OF SLEEP: _____
GLASSES OF WATER FOR TODAY : _____

NOTES

What I have achieved Today

_____

_____

_____

_____

_____

What I need to improve next

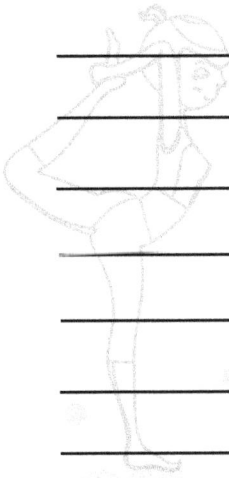

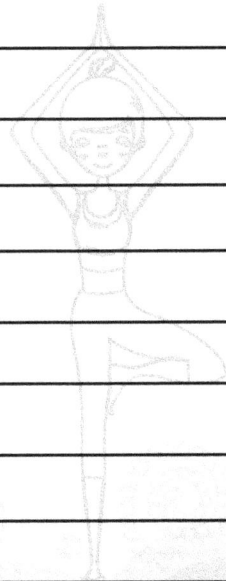

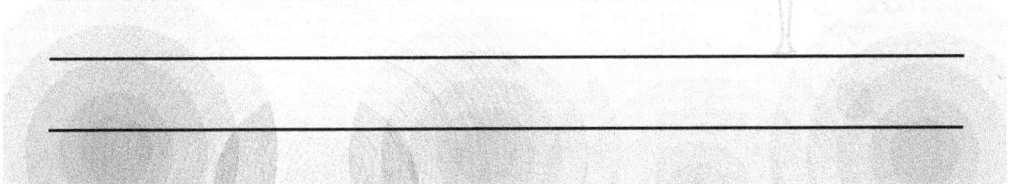

_____

_____

_____

_____

_____

_____

_____

_____

_____

_____

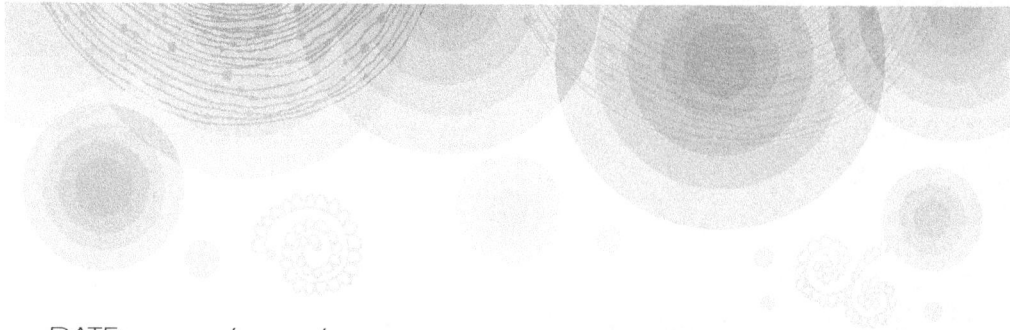

DATE: _____/_____/_____

STRENGTH TRAINING		Time Start:			Time Stop:	
EXERCISE	SET 1	SET 2	SET 3	SET 4	SET5	

CARDIO		Time Start:		Time Stop:		
EXERCISE	TIME	INTENSITY	DISTANCE	RATE	CALORIES	

NOTES

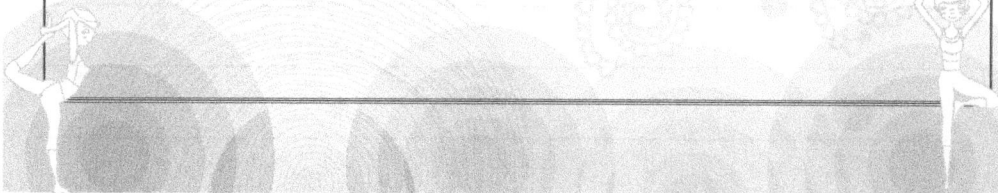

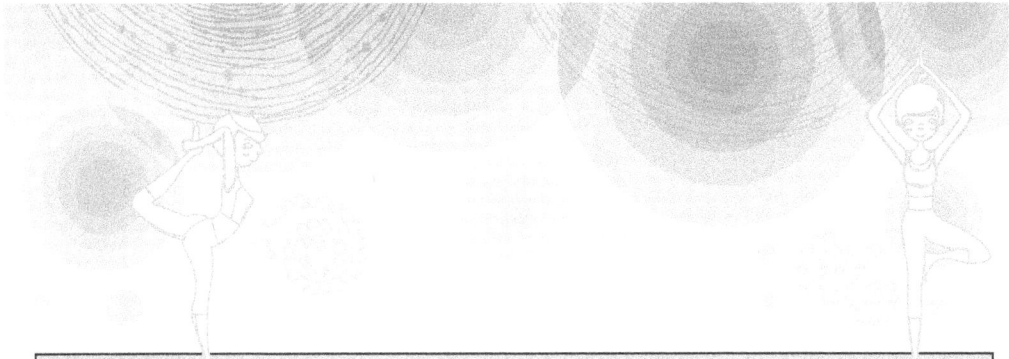

FOOD LOG

BREAKFAST	NOTES

SNACK	NOTES

LUNCH	NOTES

SNACK	NOTES

DINNER	NOTES

NUTRIENT TRACKER

	# OF SERVINGS						
GRAIN							
VEGGIES							
FRUITS							
DAIRY							
PROTEIN							
FATS							
VITAMINS							
SUGAR							

NOTES

HOURS OF SLEEP: _____

GLASSES OF WATER FOR TODAY : _____

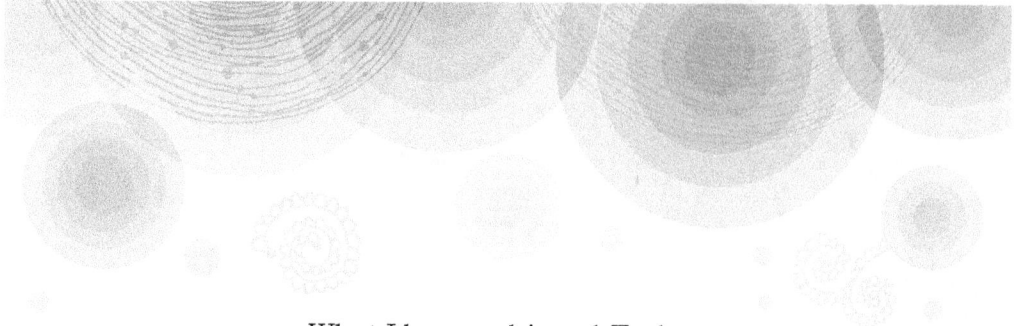

What I have achieved Today

_____

_____

_____

_____

_____

_____

What I need to improve next

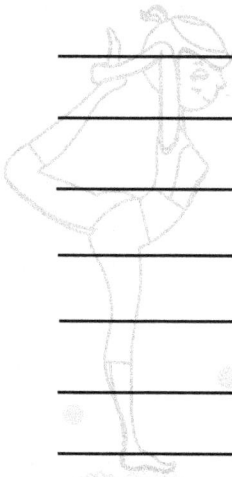

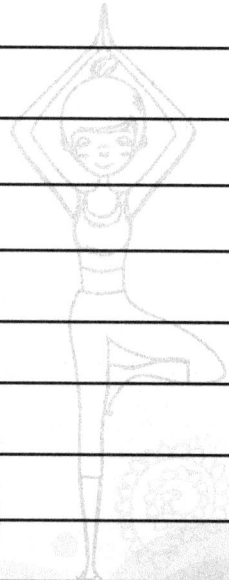

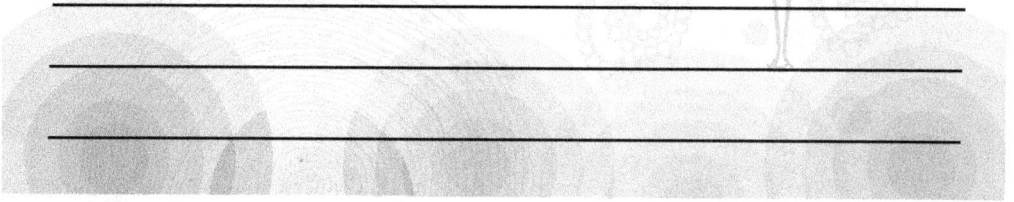

_____

_____

_____

_____

_____

_____

_____

_____

_____

DATE: _____/ _____/ _____

STRENGTH TRAINING		Time Start:			Time Stop:	
EXERCISE	SET 1	SET 2	SET 3	SET 4	SET5

CARDIO		Time Start:			Time Stop:	
EXERCISE	TIME	INTENSITY	DISTANCE	RATE	CALORIES

NOTES

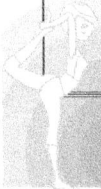
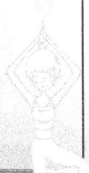

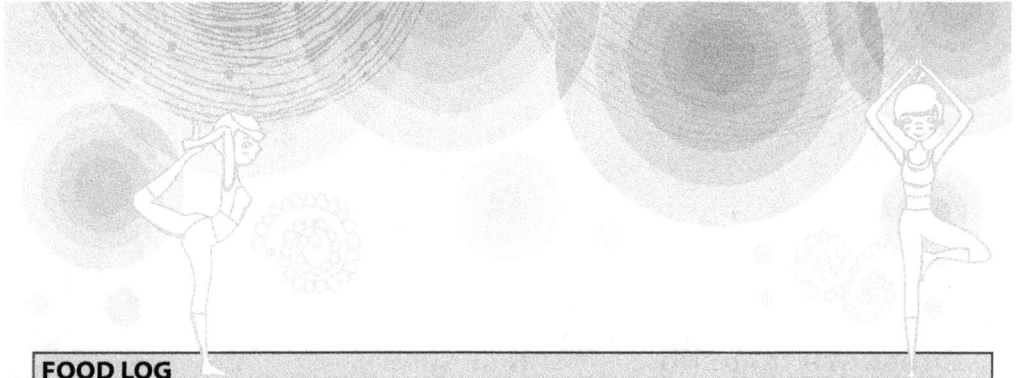

FOOD LOG

BREAKFAST	NOTES

SNACK	NOTES

LUNCH	NOTES

SNACK	NOTES

DINNER	NOTES

NUTRIENT TRACKER

	# OF SERVINGS						
GRAIN							
VEGGIES							
FRUITS							
DAIRY							
PROTEIN							
FATS							
VITAMINS							
SUGAR							

NOTES

HOURS OF SLEEP: _____

GLASSES OF WATER FOR TODAY : _____

What I have achieved Today

_____

_____

_____

_____

_____

_____

What I need to improve next

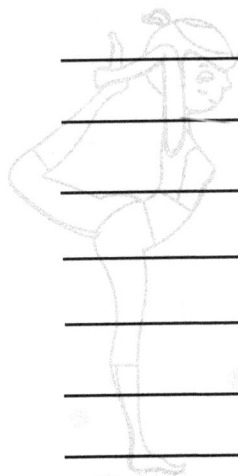

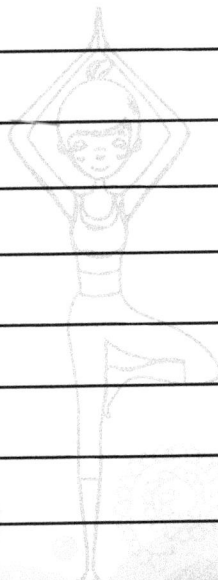

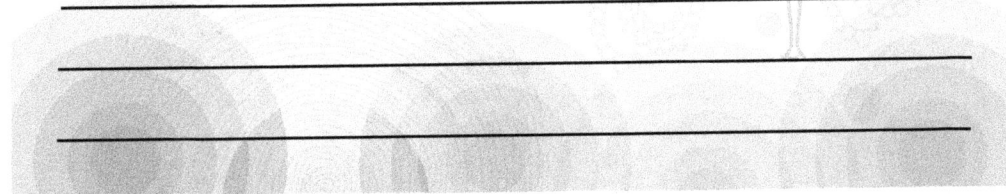

_____

_____

_____

_____

_____

_____

_____

_____

_____

_____

_____

_____

DATE: _____/_____/_____

STRENGTH TRAINING		Time Start:		Time Stop:		
EXERCISE	SET 1	SET 2	SET 3	SET 4	SET5

CARDIO		Time Start:		Time Stop:		
EXERCISE	TIME	INTENSITY	DISTANCE	RATE	CALORIES

NOTES

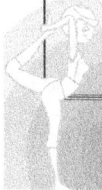
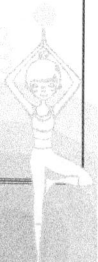

FOOD LOG

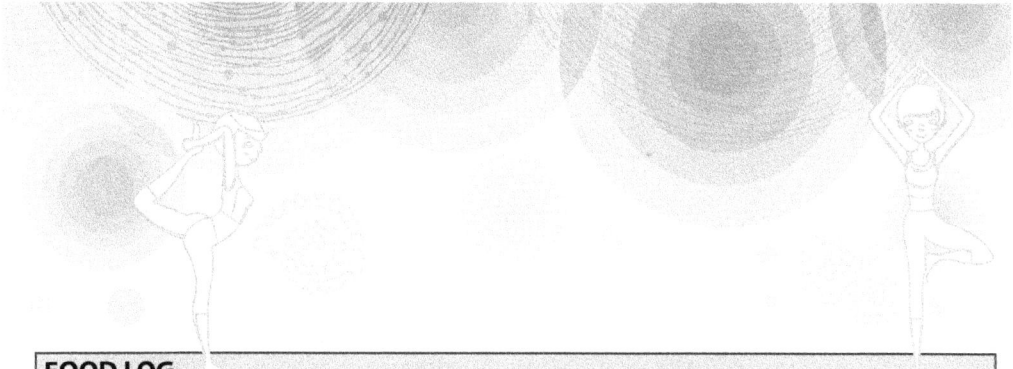

BREAKFAST	NOTES
SNACK	NOTES
LUNCH	NOTES
SNACK	NOTES
DINNER	NOTES

NUTRIENT TRACKER

	# OF SERVINGS						
GRAIN							
VEGGIES							
FRUITS							
DAIRY							
PROTEIN							
FATS							
VITAMINS							
SUGAR							

NOTES

HOURS OF SLEEP: _____

GLASSES OF WATER FOR TODAY : _____

What I have achieved Today

_____

_____

_____

_____

_____

What I need to improve next

_____

_____

_____

_____

_____

_____

_____

_____

DATE: _____/_____/_____

STRENGTH TRAINING	Time Start:		Time Stop:		
EXERCISE	SET 1	SET 2	SET 3	SET 4	SET5

CARDIO	Time Start:		Time Stop:		
EXERCISE	TIME	INTENSITY	DISTANCE	RATE	CALORIES

NOTES

www.ingramcontent.com/pod-product-compliance
Lightning Source LLC
Chambersburg PA
CBHW081419270326
41931CB00015B/3340